Vestibular Migraine in Children and Adolescents: An overview

Jeyasakthy Saniasiaya
Editor

Vestibular Migraine in Children and Adolescents: An overview

Springer

Editor
Jeyasakthy Saniasiaya
Department of Otorhinolaryngology,
Faculty of Medicine, Universiti Malaya
Kuala Lumpur, Wilayah Persekutuan Kuala Lumpur
Malaysia

ISBN 978-981-96-2166-8 ISBN 978-981-96-2167-5 (eBook)
https://doi.org/10.1007/978-981-96-2167-5

This Springer imprint is published by the registered company Springer Nature Singapore Pte Ltd.
The registered company address is: 152 Beach Road, #21-01/04 Gateway East, Singapore 189721, Singapore

Acknowledgement

I humbly express my deepest gratitude to all my mentors for all the guidance and encouragement that I have continuously received throughout my career.

To my beloved husband Dr. Prakashrao Appareo: You are my world. No words can express how much your support, love, and strength means to me.

To my parents, my brother, my parents-in-law, and family: Thank you for your love, and patience. Your unwavering support, love and encouragement have been the foundation of my journey. I am forever grateful for your sacrifices and guidance, which have made this endeavor possible.

To my co-authors: Each of you has been a great mentor to me, and I am truly humbled by your willingness to contribute to this book without hesitation. Your expertise and guidance have been invaluable in shaping this project, and I am deeply grateful for your support in advancing the field of paediatric vestibular research and care.

Jeyasakthy Saniasiaya

Contents

Contributors

Jacob R. Brodsky, MD, FACS, FAAP Department of Otolaryngology and Communication Enhancement, Boston Children's Hospital, Harvard Medical School, Boston, MA, USA

Sharon L. Cushing, MD, MSc, FRCSC Department of Otolaryngology—Head & Neck Surgery, University of Toronto, The Hospital for Sick Children, Toronto, ON, Canada

Soumit Dasgupta, MBBS, DLO, MS, FRCS, MSc School of Medical and Health Sciences, University of Liverpool, Liverpool, UK
School of Psychological Sciences, University of Manchester, Manchester, UK
Paediatric Audiology, Alder Hey Children's NHS Foundation Trust, Liverpool, UK

Carolyn M. Jenks, MD Department of Otolaryngology—Head and Neck Surgery, Johns Hopkins University, Baltimore, MD, USA

Jeyanthi Kulasegarah, BCh, MB, BAO, FRCS ORLHNS, MD Department of Otorhinolaryngology, Faculty of Medicine, Universiti Malaya, Kuala Lumpur, Wilayah Persekutuan Kuala Lumpur, Malaysia

Narayanan Prepageran, MBBS, MS ORL, FRCS (Edin) Department of Otorhinolaryngology, Faculty of Medicine, Universiti Malaya, Kuala Lumpur, Wilayah Persekutuan Kuala Lumpur, Malaysia

Sudhira A. B. Ratnayake, MBBS, MRCS Ed, DO-HNS, MSc School of Medicine, Faculty of Health and Life Sciences, University of Liverpool, Liverpool, UK
Postgraduate School of Medicine, NHS England, North West, UK
Department of Audio-Vestibular Medicine & Audiology, Alder Hey Children's NHS Foundation Trust, Liverpool, UK

Jeyasakthy Saniasiaya, MD, MMED ORL-HNS, FEBEORLHNS Department of Otorhinolaryngology, Faculty of Medicine, Universiti Malayas, Kuala Lumpur, Wilayah Persekutuan Kuala Lumpur, Malaysia

Josine Widdershoven, MD, PhD Department of Otorhinolaryngology, Maastricht University Medical Center, Maastricht, The Netherlands
Department of Otorhinolaryngology, Antwerp University Hospital, Antwerp, Belgium

Vestibular Migraine in Children: What Do We Know

1

Jeyasakthy Saniasiaya and Sharon L. Cushing

1.1 Introduction

Vestibular medicine is a well-established field among adults, with extensive data and research worldwide. Vestibular disorders in children and adolescents have only gained attention over the past decade, with limited research and publications on this topic. The prevalence of vestibular disorders among children has been reported to be between 0.7% and 15% [1, 2], although recent reports suggest that the incidence may actually be higher [3].

Difficulty verbalising symptoms, short-lived nature, rapid compensation, and lack of awareness among parents and children result in vestibular disorders being under-recognised in children. Although paediatric vestibular medicine is a growing field, a lack of expertise and trained specialists across the globe has contributed to affected children being missed and overlooked. The lack of biomarkers or diagnostic tools to diagnose this condition also contributes to the paucity of data.

VM is the most common cause of dizziness in the adult population [4, 5]. Interestingly, VM has also been found to be the most common cause of dizziness in children and adolescence [2, 6–9]. VM can be defined as episodic vertigo that accompanies migrainous headaches, although vertigo or headache may occur independently. The fundamental tool in diagnosing VM is clinical history.

J. Saniasiaya (✉)
Department of Otorhinolaryngology, Faculty of Medicine, Universiti Malaya, Kuala Lumpur, Wilayah Persekutuan Kuala Lumpur, Malaysia
e-mail: jeyasakthy@um.edu.my

S. L. Cushing
Department of Otolaryngology—Head & Neck Surgery, University of Toronto, The Hospital for Sick Children, Toronto, ON, Canada
e-mail: sharon.cushing@sickkids.ca

J. Saniasiaya (ed.), *Vestibular Migraine in Children and Adolescents: An overview*, https://doi.org/10.1007/978-981-96-2167-5_1

Over the past decade, different terms have been proposed to describe VM, including vertiginous migraine, migrainous vertigo, migraine-related dizziness, migraine with prominent vertigo, migraine-related vestibulopathy, migraine-associated dizziness, benign recurrent vertigo, and benign paroxysmal vertigo. Kayan and Hood introduced this condition in 1984, encompassing headache, vertigo, and visual phenomena [10]. However, Dieterich and Brandt coined the term vestibular migraine in 1999, which describes vestibular symptoms caused by migraine [4].

1.2 History

The understanding of vestibular migraine (VM) dates back to the Hippocrates era. According to the Hippocratic collection, vertigo was considered a condition affecting the head that can be accompanied by a throbbing headache [11]. Subsequently, numerous observations with regard to the link between migraine and vertigo were made by numerous physicians [12–15]. However, the association between vertigo and migraine or headache probably gained attention following Shelby and Lance's large series publication, whereby 33% of the included 500 patients with migraine, termed vascular headache, were reported to have vertigo [16]. Later, in 1961, Bickerstaff described basilar-type migraine or basilar artery migraine [17].

1.2.1 Prevalence and Epidemiology

The majority of the earlier epidemiological studies involving the paediatric population have pooled dizziness and imbalance [2, 18] together and also have included all types of dizziness symptoms, including the nonvestibular-related types of dizziness, making it difficult to estimate the exact prevalence or incidence of symptoms. The one-year prevalence of dizziness and balance conditions, as reported in a population-based study in the United States in children between 3 and 17 years, was 5.6% with mean [SD] age = 10.3 [4.4] years (Brodsky et al., 2020) [1].

The exact prevalence of VM in children remains unknown as there is no population-based data on the prevalence of VM in children and adolescents. In addition to that, varying diagnostic criteria and terms used have contributed to the discrepancy in the incidence of VM in children and adolescents. Based on the published literature worldwide, the incidence of VM or migraine-related vertigo in children and adolescents is reported to be between 17.6% and 58% [9, 19–23].

1.3 Clinical Manifestation and Diagnostic Criteria

Unlike in adults, diagnosing VM in children and adolescents remains a challenge. The clinical manifestation of VM can vary, although, in younger children, the symptoms are shorter and better tolerated. The inability to verbalise symptoms and lack of understanding and awareness of what is happening pose a dilemma in diagnosis.

Over the past decade, several criteria have been published to aid in diagnosing VM, albeit mostly involving the adult population. Neuhauser et al. formulated the first diagnostic criteria [24]. Subsequently, the Committee for Classification of Vestibular Disorders of the Bárány Society and the Migraine Classification Subcommittee of the International Headache Society (IHS) developed diagnostic criteria for VM, which proposed that at least five episodes of vestibular symptoms are required in order to diagnose VM. The committee introduced a new criterion, 'probable vestibular migraine', if the patient is found to have no history of migraine or its features are absent during the vestibular episodes [25].

The recent consensus document of the Classification Committee of Vestibular Disorders of the Barany Society and the International Headache Society in 2021 has proposed classifying VM in children into three groups: vestibular migraine of childhood, probable vestibular migraine of childhood, and recurrent vertigo of childhood according to the nature, duration of symptoms, and accompanying conditions [6]. These new criteria appear to represent the paediatric population (age under 18 years) and represent the spectrum of clinical presentations that is more relevant to children [6].

Benign paroxysmal vertigo of childhood was previously described as a separate entity, with a reported prevalence of 3% [2, 22, 26]. Benign paroxysmal vertigo was initially described as an early manifestation of migraine in children [26, 27]. Historically described by Basser in 1964, benign paroxysmal vertigo of childhood entails the presence of recurrent spontaneous attacks of vertigo accompanied by frightfulness, pallor, vomiting, ataxia, imbalance, and nystagmus [28]. Benign paroxysmal vertigo of childhood was described as a condition that begins before age 4 and resolves between the ages of 8 and 10 in an otherwise healthy child [28]. Children diagnosed with benign paroxysmal vertigo of childhood were reported to develop VM in adulthood later, although there is still a lack of sufficient data on this. Parallel to this, as there is no concrete evidence to prove benign paroxysmal vertigo of childhood to be a separate entity or a part of VM, the recent consensus document of the Classification Committee of Vestibular Disorders of the Barany Society and the International Headache Society has decided to replace benign paroxysmal vertigo of childhood with recurrent vertigo of childhood [6].

1.4 Risk Factors

1.4.1 Age

The age of onset of VM was reported to vary. In a recent study by Teggi et al., it was reported that the age of onset of vertigo was earlier in children in the RVC (range 5–12), followed by pVMC (range 9–17) and VMC (11–17) [27]. In another study by Zhang et al., the age of the cohort with VM was 10.7 ± 2.9 (range: 6–17) years [29]. A recent systematic review of VM among children reported that the median age of the included children was 10.9 years [30].

1.4.2 Race

Data on racial predisposition among children with VM remains unknown due to the lack of reported studies as well as due to the non-standardised approach to categorising VM. The population-based studies reported a higher prevalence of VM among the African-American population or Europeans in comparison to those of Asian descent, suggesting a possible genetic contribution. Yet, it is worth mentioning that paediatric vestibular services have only recently been established across the Asian continent, which could contribute to biased data [31].

1.4.3 Gender

VM is found to affect female children more than males, notably among adolescents. A recent systematic review reported a higher female preponderance of 62.3% among children and adolescents with VM [median age: 10.9] [30]. A large-population-based study among children conducted in the United States demonstrated that females with frequent headaches/migraine were found to have a higher prevalence of dizziness and balance conditions, suggesting a possibility of VM among females [32]. Another population-based study by Filippopulos et al. demonstrated that female students are at 1.17 times higher risk of developing vertigo than male students [33]. Female sex has also been associated with vertigo across various studies on vestibular conditions, notably in adolescence [34–36]. Previous reports have suggested that the higher risk of vestibular conditions in female adolescents was postulated to be secondary to autonomic integrity disturbance [37].

Akin to that, in the adult population, female patients have been found to be over-represented in vestibular disorders, especially in VM [31]. Based on the largest epidemiological study involving 70,315,919, it was found that female patients were more frequently affected by dizziness and vertigo, irrespective of age and specific cause [38]. It is worth noting that, up to the age of 14, the prevalence of vestibular conditions was found to be similar [38].

1.4.4 Family History

A family history of migraine has been found to be a notable risk factor for VM among children [9, 39–43]. A recent systematic review demonstrated that 75.65% of children with VM were found to have a family history of migraine. Akin to that, children with a familial history of migraine were more prone to be classified into the VMC group in comparison to other subtypes: probable VMC or RVC [44]. Nonetheless, a family history of migraine involving first-degree relatives reported a twofold rise in the risk of developing VM [26].

1.4.5 Genetic Inheritance

Although a family history of migraine supports the possibility of genetic origin, it does not appear to follow the Mendelian inheritance pattern. Nonetheless, the familial clustering observed supports the role of genetic contribution [45]. An autosomal dominant inheritance with moderate to high penetrance has been reported, albeit no mutations have been found [46, 47]. Several loci segregating VM were found through linkage analysis among affected family members in 22q12 [48] and 5q35 [49], which suggests that individuals with VM could have the polygenic type of inheritance.

Additionally, experts have found several genes to be associated with a subset of migraine, such as familial hemiplegic migraine, including FHM1, the CACNA1A gene on chromosome 19; FHM2, the ATP1A2 gene on chromosome 1; and FHM3, the SCN1A gene on chromosome 2.

1.4.6 Lifestyle

It is worth noting here that most of the reported data on the effect of poor lifestyle revolve around children and adolescents with migraine, following the paucity of research on children with VM. Unhealthy lifestyles such as fast food, stress, poor sleep, and a sedentary lifestyle are risk factors for VM in children.

1.4.7 Associated Conditions with VM

Several conditions, such as motion sickness, Meniere's disease, benign positional postural vertigo, and somatoform, have been associated with VM (further discussed in later chapter).

Reports of overlapping symptoms between VM and Meniere's disease have been widely discussed, including in children [50]. 11.5% of included children with VM were reported to also have BPPV in a systematic review [41, 42]. Gedik Soyuce et al. reported that children with VM are susceptible to recurrent BPPV attacks, as 94% of the children in their series with recurrent BPPV were found to have VM [41]. This is in contradiction to reports of a much lower prevalence of BPPV generally in the paediatric population compared to adults, with concussion being the most common predictor in children who develop BPPV [51].

Children, notably adolescents, were reported to be susceptible to developing somatoform vertigo (aka functional neurologic disorder). It is postulated that perception and regulation of emotions share the same network of afferent loops in the brainstem and sensorimotor integration, resulting in mood imbalance and anxiety among children with VM [52].

1.4.8 Motion Sickness

A review on VM in children demonstrated motion sickness as a risk factor for VM [39, 41, 42].

1.5 Management

Most of the treatment of VM in children and adolescents has been adopted from the adult population as well as studies and data from paediatric migraine [30]. VM can be addressed using both pharmacological and non-pharmacological treatment. Pharmacological treatment includes abortive treatment and prophylactic treatment. To date, due to the lack of a multicentre, large prospective study, the long-term outcome in children and adolescents with VM remains unknown.

1.6 Why VM Needs to Be Addressed Early in Children and Adolescents?

Although there are reports that claim that children possess immense neural plasticity as well as the ability to compensate faster for deficits and disorders, it must also be considered that the presence and lack of treatment of such disorders may impact a child's development in a manner that need not be considered in the adult population. It is prudent to consider that children with vestibular conditions, including VM, may suffer numerous detrimental effects, including delay in gross-motor function, cognitive and learning disability, as well as psychosocial, behavioural, and emotional difficulties [53]. Early recognition and management will optimise both development and quality of life.

1.7 Conclusion

VM is the most common vestibular condition in children and adolescents. History and diagnostic criteria remain the core of diagnosing this condition with auxiliary investigations such as oto-neurological and imaging aimed at excluding other conditions. Great strides and measures to continually study this condition are warranted to better understand this entity to aid in its management.

References

1. Brodsky JR, Lipson S, Bhattacharyya N. Prevalence of pediatric dizziness and imbalance in the United States. Otolaryngol Head Neck Surg. 2020;162:241–7.
2. Gioacchini FM, Alicandri-Ciufelli M, Kaleci S, Magliulo G, Re M. Prevalence and diagnosis of vestibular disorders in children: a review. Int J Pediatr Otorhinolaryngol. 2014;78(5):718–24.

3. Saniasiaya J, Islam MA, Salim R. The global prevalence of vestibular dysfunction in children and adolescents: a systematic review and meta-analysis. Eur Arch Otorrinolaringol. 2023;280(6):2663–74.
4. Dieterich M, Brandt T. Episodic vertigo related to migraine (90 cases): vestibular migraine? J Neurol. 1999;246(10):883–92.
5. Neuhauser HK, Radtke A, von Brevern M, Feldmann M, Lezius F, Ziese T, et al. Migrainous vertigo: prevalence and impact on quality of life. Neurology. 2006;67(6):1028–33.
6. van de Berg R, Widdershoven J, Bisdorff A, et al. Vestibular migraine of childhood and recurrent vertigo of childhood: diagnostic criteria consensus document of the committee for the classification of vestibular disorders of the Bárány Society and the International Headache Society. J Vestib Res. 2021;31(1):1–9.
7. Devaraja K. Vertigo in children; a narrative review of the various causes and their management. Int J Pediatr Otorhinolaryngol. 2018;111:32–8.
8. Jahn K, Langhagen T, Schroeder AS, Heinen F. Vertigo and dizziness in childhood—update on diagnosis and treatment. Neuropediatrics. 2011;42(4):129–34.
9. Batu ED, Anlar B, Topçu M, Turanlı G, Aysun S. Vertigo in childhood: a retrospective series of 100 children. Eur J Paediatr Neurol. 2015;19(2):226–32.
10. Kayan A, Hood JD. Neuro-otological manifestations of migraine. Brain. 1984;107(Pt 4):1123–42.
11. Potter P. Hippocrates, vol. V. Cambridge: Harvard University Press; 1988. p. 196–7.
12. Boenheim F. Über familiare Hemicrania vestibularis. Neurol Zentralbl. 1917;36:226–9.
13. Heveroch J. La migraine vestibulaire. Rev Neurol. 1925;33:925–9.
14. Symonds CP. Vertigo. Postgrad Med J. 1926;1:63–5.
15. Richter H. Die Migrane Handbuch der Neurologie. Berlin: Springer; 1935. p. 166–245.
16. Selby G, Lance JW. Observations on 500 cases of migraine and allied vascular headache. J Neurol Neurosurg Psychiatry. 1960;23:23–32.
17. Bickerstaff ER. Basilar artery migraine. Lancet. 1961;227:15–7.
18. O'Reilly RC, Greywoode J, Morlet T, et al. Comprehensive vestibular and balance testing in the dizzy pediatric population. Otolaryngol Head Neck Surg. 2011;144:142–8.
19. Szirmai A. Vestibular disorders in childhood and adolescents. Eur Arch Otorrinolaringol. 2010;267(11):1801–4.
20. Niemensivu R, Kentala E, Wiener-Vacher S, Pyykko I. Evaluation of vertiginous children. Eur Arch Otorrinolaringol. 2007;264(10):1129–35.
21. Wiener-Vacher SR. Vestibular disorders in children. Int J Audiol. 2008;47(9):578–83.
22. Balatsouras DG, Kaberos A, Assimakopoulos D, Katotomichelakis M, Economou NC, Korres SG. Etiology of vertigo in children. Int J Pediatr Otorhinolaryngol. 2007;71(3):487–94.
23. Brodsky JR, Cusick BA, Zhou G. Evaluation and management of vestibular migraine in children: experience from a pediatric vestibular clinic. Eur J Paediatr Neurol. 2016;20(1):85–92. The first report on the management of VM, according to the current diagnostic criteria, in children
24. Neuhauser HK, Lempert T. Diagnostic criteria for migrainous vertigo. Acta Otolaryngol. 2005;125(11):1247–8.
25. Lempert T, Olesen J, Furman J, Waterston J, Seemungal B, Carey J, et al. Vestibular migraine: diagnostic criteria. J Vestib Res. 2012;22(4):167–72. The consensus document providing the officially accepted diagnostic criteria for VM
26. Abu-Arafeh I, Russell G. Paroxysmal vertigo as a migraine equivalent in children: a population-based study. Cephalalgia. 1995;15(1):22–4.
27. Teggi R, Colombo B, Albera R, et al. Clinical features, familial history, and migraine precursors in patients with definite vestibular migraine: the VM-phenotypes projects. Headache. 2018;58:534–44.
28. Basser LS. Benign paroxysmal vertigo of childhood. (a variety of vestibular neuronitis). Brain. 1964;87:141–52.
29. Zhang F, Shen J, Zhu Q, Wang L, Ma X, He B, Yang Y, Wang W, Chen X, Zhang Q, Jin Y, Duan M, Chen J, Yang J. Evaluating children with vestibular migraine through vestibular test bat-

tery: a cross-sectional investigation. Front Neurol. 2022;13:997217. https://doi.org/10.3389/fneur.2022.997217. PMID: 36388219; PMCID: PMC9659754

30. Saniasiaya J, Salim R. Characteristics and diagnostic approach of vestibular migraine in children and adolescents: a systematic review. Auris Nasus Larynx. 2023;50(2):218–27. https://doi.org/10.1016/j.anl.2022.06.007.
31. Formeister EJ, Rizk HG, Kohn MA, Sharon JD. The epidemiology of vestibular migraine: a population-based survey study. Otol Neurotol. 2018;39(8):1037–44.
32. Li CM, Hoffman HJ, Ward BK, Cohen HS, Rine RM. Epidemiology of dizziness and balance problems in children in the United States: a population-based study. J Pediatr. 2016;171:240–7.e3. Most recent and large epidemiological report on dizziness and vertigo in childhood
33. Filippopulos FM, Albers L, Straube A, et al. Vertigo and dizziness in adolescents: risk factors and their population attributable risk. PLoS One. 2017;12(11):e0187819.
34. Sloane P. Dizziness in primary care. Results from the National Ambulatory Medical Care Survey. J Fam Pract. 1989;29(1):33–8. pmid:2738548
35. Aggarwal N, Bennett D, Bienias J, Mendes DLC, Morris M, Evans D. The prevalence of dizziness and its association with functional disability in a biracial community population. J Gerontol A Biol Sci Med Sci. 2000;55(5):M288. pmid:10819319
36. Neuhauser HK. Epidemiology of vertigo. Curr Opin Neurol. 2007;20(1):40–6. pmid:17215687
37. Fu Q, Witkowski S, Okazaki K, Levine BD. Effects of gender and hypovolemia on sympathetic neural responses to orthostatic stress. Am J Phys. 2005;289:R109–R16.
38. Hülse R, Biesdorf A, Hörmann K, et al. Peripheral vestibular disorders: an epidemiologic survey in 70 million individuals. Otol Neurotol. 2019;40(1):88–95.
39. Weisleder P, Fife TD. Dizziness and headache: a common association in children and adolescents. J Child Neurol. 2001;16:727–30.
40. Langhagen T, Lehrer N, Borggraefe I, Heinen F, Jahn K. Vestibular migraine in children and adolescents: clinical findings and laboratory tests. Front Neurol. 2015;5:292.
41. Gedik-Soyuyuce O, Gence-Gumus Z, Ozdilek A, Ada M, Korkut N. Vestibular disorders in children: a retrospective analysis of vestibular function test findings. Int J Pediatr Otorhinolaryngol. 2021;146:110751.
42. Marcelli V, Furia T, Marciano E. Vestibular pathways involvement in children with migraine: a neuro-otological study. Headache. 2010;50:71–6.
43. Božanić Urbančič N, Vozel D, Kordiš Š, Hribar M, Urbančič J, Battelino S. Indicators of pediatric peripheral vestibular disorder: a retrospective study in a tertiary referral center. Int J Pediatr Otorhinolaryngol. 2022;159:111221.
44. Teggi R, Colombo B, Familiari M, Cangiano I, Bussi M, Filippi M. Phenotypes, bedside examination, and video head impulse test in vestibular migraine of childhood compared with probable vestibular migraine and recurrent vertigo in childhood. Front Pediatr. 2023;11:1152928.
45. Espinosa-Sanchez JM, Lopez-Escamez JA. New insights into pathophysiology of vestibular migraine. Front Neurol. 2015;6:12.
46. von Brevern M, Ta N, Shankar A, et al. Migrainous vertigo: mutation analysis of the candidate genes CACNA1A, ATP1A2, SCN1A, and CACNB4. Headache. 2006;46(7):1136–41. https://doi.org/10.1111/j.1526-4610.2006.00504.x.
47. Kim JS, Yue Q, Jen JC, Nelson SF, Baloh RW. Familial migraine with vertigo: no mutations found in CACNA1A. Am J Med Genet. 1998;79(2):148–51.
48. Lee H, Jen JC, Wang H, et al. A genome-wide linkage scan of familial benign recurrent vertigo: linkage to 22q12 with evidence of heterogeneity. Hum Mol Genet. 2006;15(2):251–8.
49. Bahmad F Jr, DePalma SR, Merchant SN, et al. Locus for familial migrainous vertigo disease maps to chromosome 5q35. Ann Otol Rhinol Laryngol. 2009;118(9):670–6.
50. Abouzari M, Abiri A, Djalilian HR. Successful treatment of a child with definite Meniere's disease with the migraine regimen. Am J Otolaryngol. 2019;40(3):440–2. https://doi.org/10.1016/j.amjoto.2019.02.004. Epub 2019 Feb 18. PMID: 30803806; PMCID: PMC8041434

51. Wang A, Zhou G, Kawai K, O'Brien M, Shearer AE, Brodsky JR. Benign paroxysmal positional vertigo in children and adolescents with concussion. Sports Health. 2021;13(4):380–6. https://doi.org/10.1177/1941738120970515.
52. Langhagen T, Schroeder AS, Rettinger N, Borggraefe I, Jahn K. Migraine-related vertigo and somatoform vertigo frequently occur in children and are often associated. Neuropediatrics. 2013;44:55–8.
53. Reale L, Guarnera M, Grillo C, Maiolino L, Ruta L, Mazzone L. Psychological assessment in children and adolescents with benign paroxysmal vertigo. Brain and Development. 2011;33(2):125–30. https://doi.org/10.1016/j.braindev.2010.03.006.

Pathogenesis of Vestibular Migraine in Children

2

Soumit Dasgupta

2.1 Introduction

2.1.1 Definition of Migraine

Migraine is a neurological disorder that is traditionally characterised by a throbbing or pulsatile headache, episodic in nature and occasionally self-limiting. Headache is a nonspecific symptom and can occur in a wide variety of physical and mental disorders. The headache in classical migraine follows a pattern with autonomic symptoms that have led to define it as a definite neurological disorder. The International Classification of Headache Disorders 3 (ICHD 3) lists migraine with aura, migraine without aura (including hemiplegic migraine, chronic migraine), complications of migraine (including status migrainous, migrainous infarction, persistent aura triggered seizure and persistent aura without infarction), probable migraine, episodic syndromes associated with migraine (including cyclical vomiting, abdominal migraine, benign paroxysmal vertigo and benign spasmodic torticollis) [1]. Migrainous spells are often but not invariably precipitated by a trigger, e.g. dehydration, intense physical activities, challenging sensory environments, motion, menstruation cycles, stress and anxiety, sleep deprivation and some food products like chocolate, cheese, red wine, red meat, alcohol and citrus fruits.

S. Dasgupta (✉)
Paediatric Audiology, Alder Hey Children's NHS Foundation Trust, Liverpool, UK

School of Medical and Health Sciences, University of Liverpool, Liverpool, UK

School of Psychological Sciences, University of Manchester, Manchester, UK
e-mail: soumit.dasgupta@alderhey.nhs.uk

J. Saniasiaya (ed.), *Vestibular Migraine in Children and Adolescents: An overview*, https://doi.org/10.1007/978-981-96-2167-5_2

2.1.2 History

In antiquity, unilateral headache first finds mention in the Ebers papyrus in circa 3500 BC. Interestingly, the papyrus also describes dizziness with the headache as well alluding to a vestibular migraine that will be eventually discovered several millennia later [2]. Hippocrates was the first physician to describe visual disturbances with the headache and the headache relieved by vomiting. Aretaeus of Cappadocia, Galen, Rhazes and Gariopontus in ancient Greece and Rome and medieval Arabia described migraine. They were also pioneers in vestibular pathology, which was unknown during those times and manifested as dizziness [2]. Lieving in 1873 was the first in modern times to associate vertigo with migraine [3], later thought to be a prodromal feature of classical migraine, especially by Bickerstaff in 1961 who defined basilar artery migraine with vertigo, visual disturbances and ataxia as the prodrome [4]. Therefore, right from ancient times, migraine and vestibular symptoms were often described hand in hand.

2.1.3 Vestibular Migraine (VM)

The very first time in modern times where migraine of the vestibular system was thought of as a different entity from a classical brain migraine was in the seminal paper by Kayan and Hood in 1984 [5]. They identified that in a cohort of migraine patients with vestibular symptoms, about 77.5% presented with persistent and objective vestibular derangements as compared to only about 59% in an unselected general migraine group. This led them to propose that these vestibular symptoms were due to involvement of the vertebrobasilar territory in migraine that supplies the labyrinthine apparatus and therefore behaved differently from classical migraine. The idea was subsequently picked up by Neuehauser and Lempert in 2004 who for the first time defined a migrainous vertigo (MV) as a separate entity to classical migraine where the cardinal symptom of the latter, i.e. a headache, was replaced by the classical vestibular symptom of vertigo in the former [6]. Research followed and in 2012, the Barany Society published the first diagnostic criteria for vestibular migraine (VM) that was updated in 2022 [7]. The ICHD 3 recognised this and included the entity in their classification in 2018 [1].

The classification of VM and its variants is less clear in children than in adults. A condition was described called benign positional vertigo in childhood (BPVC). This was first proposed by Basser in 1964, where children presenting with episodic vertiginous symptoms mimicked an acute vestibular neuritis phenotype, yet were distinct from it [8]. The symptoms merged with migrainous symptoms. Further reports led to establishing the condition as BPVC and it was proposed that this was a migraine variant [9]. In a review article published in 2004, it was inferred that the evidence for BPVC as a migraine variant was quite compelling [10]. The Barany criteria for childhood vestibular migraine were published in 2021 that merged BPVC with a broader umbrella of vestibular migraine in childhood [11]. This is because the committee formulating the guidelines deemed that paroxysms by definition last for seconds, whilst VM spells in children last for minutes to hours. There is a distinct clinical entity called vestibular paroxysmia (VP) that has an entirely different pathogenesis than VM. Therefore, for a symptom criteria-based diagnosis, overlapping of symptoms between 2 conditions does generate some ambiguity and a diagnostic conundrum. However, it must be borne in mind that a paroxysm can last for minutes (e.g. in multiple sclerosis) and a BPVC attack can last for seconds. Therefore, the term BPVC should be retained for children with VM under the age of 4 years where the attacks last only for seconds. From age 4, the VM attacks show characteristics as given in the Barany criteria when the durations of spells get longer.

2.1.4 VM Epidemiology and Phenotype in Children

Vestibular migraine on all counts is the commonest cause for dizziness in children accounting up to 25% of children presenting with dizziness [12–14]. In the adult population, it accounts for 4–10% of adult dizziness [15]. Therefore, it is more common in children than in adults due to reasons that can be explained by the differences in brain metabolism and cerebral plasticity given in the next sections.

The diagnosis of VM in children is a careful clinical decision and might not be as clear cut as found in adults. This is because it is often quite difficult to elicit a history from young children and VM is a diagnosis based on anamnesis. Vestibular behaviour in children as observed by their parents/carers is a sensitive indicator of vestibular pathology. In many instances, indirect history, such as change of facial expression, sudden drop attacks and closure of eyes during episodes are pivotal to make a diagnosis.

The Barany criteria for childhood VM do not factor in the difficulties faced in eliciting VM history from children. It works for those children who can narrate a personal history, e.g. teenagers. Diagnosing a VM in children from the diagnostic criteria alone might not be enough [14] and rigidity and lack of flexibility in applying the criteria are not recommended. Often the children do not fulfil the criteria and their phenotypes become atypical. The phenotype as propounded by the Barany criteria might be different in different children. Thus, diagnosis of VM in children is a highly skilled process requiring significant clinical judgement with a holistic knowledge in paediatric pathologies spanning across different organs. It has to crucially take into account the fourth criteria of diagnosis, i.e. exclusion of other causes. Indeed, a child with a VM phenotype must undergo all investigations, including full audiovestibular quantification and/or imaging.

2.2 Differences Between Adult and Child Brain Function

In order to understand the pathophysiology of vestibular migraine in children on which there is a dearth of research, it will be useful to revisit the differences in brain metabolism and cerebral plasticity. This is because of the fundamental premise that a child's brain and the vestibular organ are in states of development and show a much higher metabolic rate than in adults that can offer some protection against the VM process. These differences are important as they suggest that the manifestations of migraine and VM in children as compared to adults are not only different but also are variable determined by the age of the child. It is inappropriate to consider a child as a miniature adult as the physiology in each is different.

2.2.1 Child and Adult Brain Metabolism

In the developing brain in a child, there is a case to propose that with a dynamic evolution of metabolite secretion, further changes may bring on a migraine spell that will be different as compared to adults. Since an adult brain is not subjected to an additional high metabolic process as occurs in a developing brain, the prevalence of VM is more common in children than in adults.

It has been shown that key metabolites in the brain like N-acetylaspartate (NAA), total choline (tCho) and glutamate plus glutamine show changes throughout childhood and are likely influencing various processes and of functional brain development [16]. All these chemicals show changes in migraine [17–19]. NAA plays a role in neuronal metabolism, myelination and synthesis of N-acetylaspartylglutamate (NAAG) and continues to rise in childhood. Choline participates in myelination and declines as a child grows up.

Glutamate is an important neuroexcitatory metabolite and deserves special mention as it is directly implicated in a migrainous process. The glutamate secretion is highest around 7 years of age and then starts to decline and attains adult values in adolescence [17]. An optimal balance is achieved by glutamate inhibition. A shift of the balance to excitation has been linked with neurodevelopmental conditions like autism or attention disorders [20]. Migrainous activity in a child may result in a similar shift and explains partly the intense behavioural reaction observed in children with VM where they are unable to function socially or in school.

Another metabolite that might be important to influence migraine is taurine whose levels in childhood decline as the child grows older. Taurine participates in inhibitory neurotransmission and protecting the brain against toxic metabolites [21]. Taurine levels increase in migraine [22], probably due to the brain's innate ability to counteract the migrainous process. In a developing brain with decreasing taurine levels in a child, this has the potential to interfere the migrainous process in a different way as compared to adults.

Cerebral blood flow in children and oxygen demands are also different in children than adults. The brains of children show an increased oxygen demand and cerebral blood flow peaking at 7 years of age [23]. If migraines including vestibular migraines are attributed to a partly vascular cause, then migraines in VM in children are prone to manifest an enhanced global phenotype as compared to adults, which is indeed the case. In other words, symptomatology in children will incorporate more central features than adults like autonomic symptoms or focal neurological signs during the ictal phase, especially with balance and the psychological reaction it generates [24].

2.2.2 Child and Adult Cerebral Plasticity

It is well known that a child's brain is more plastic than the adult brain as brain substrates and brain function are still under construction. Synaptic plasticity is the most important attribute around which cerebral plasticity is centred [25]. These synapses are responsible for establishing changing neuronal circuitry and connections and essentially teaming up different parts of the brain. This activity is maximum from birth, extending into childhood, and then decelerates.

Of the two neurotransmitters, most important for synaptic connections are glutamate and gamma-aminobutyric acid (GABA), the former is excitatory and the latter inhibitory. A fine balance is achieved in the developing brain [26]. Given the derangements in glutamate excitotoxicity as seen earlier upsetting this balance, in migraine/VM in children, the system becomes more prone to changes with the migrainous process.

2.3 Pathophysiology

There is a lack of evidence regarding pathophysiology of VM in children, but there is a sizeable literature in adults. Even then, pathogenesis of migraine is unclear. It is likely that the pathophysiology of VM in adults and in children will be fundamentally similar, but the effects thereof will be different due to the difference in cerebral plasticity and metabolism as highlighted in the earlier section.

2.3.1 Vascular Pathology

Vasospasm of the internal auditory artery was proposed to generate the vertigo of migraine with an occasional sensorineural hearing loss [27]. However, this did not explain the accompanying central features of VM. Therefore, the proposal extended to include a vasospasm of the anteroinferior cerebellar artery [28]. Neurometabolite derangement especially in the trigeminovascular pathway that drives any migrainous process has been implicated for these vascular alterations. These include neurokinin, CGRP and substance P, which are released from trigeminal sensory nerves and lead to the vasospasm [29] that is discussed later.

Functional imaging has failed to demonstrate any significant intracranial vessel alterations, thereby not confirming a direct vascular pathogenetic mechanism [30] in VM.

2.3.2 Trigeminovascular System

From the annals of migraine research, there is a general consensus that the trigeminovascular system (TVS) is critically responsible for modulating the migrainous process followed by its spread affecting several other pathways in its wake [31]. Broadly, the TVS essentially consists of neurones with cell bodies in the trigeminal ganglion in the petrous part of the temporal bone with central and peripheral connections to cranial blood vessels. The ganglionic neurones end in the trigeminal nucleus in the brainstem.

The trigeminal nucleus is the largest nerve nucleus in the body and has three distinct portions. The mesencephalic nucleus (MSTN) spans across the whole of the midbrain and specifically in the caudal midbrain and the rostral pons at the region of the periaqueductal grey region next to the cerebral aqueduct that connects the third ventricle to the fourth ventricle [32]. The main sensory nucleus (MTSN) is located in the caudal pons [32]. There is also a caudal nucleus (CTN) that is located in the medulla and travels to the adjacent spinal trigeminal tract [32]. The MSTN receives its afferents from the jaw, the MTSN receives its input from the head and the face and proprioception of the jaw whilst the CTN receives tactile, nociceptive and thermal sensations and teams up with the MSTN. It is the connections of the trigeminal nuclei that are implicated in spread of migraine/VM focus.

Specifically, the TVS constitutes pseudounipolar nociceptive ganglion of the trigemino-cervical complex (TCC) as mentioned above, including the CTN that innervates the meninges and the cranial blood vessels, receiving its first-order neuron from the ophthalmic division of the trigeminal nerve [32]. The second-order neurons ascend through the quintothalamic tract and connect to the contralateral ventroposteromedial (VPM) and the posterior thalamic nuclei that terminate in the somatosensory cortex in the temporal, parietal, insular and cingulate cortical regions [33] as the third-order neurones. Reciprocal connections to brainstem centres involved in the processing of nociceptive information include the rostral ventromedial medulla, the nucleus raphe magnus, the ventrolateral periaqueductal grey and the nociceptive areas of the posterior hypothalamus [34]. The TCC is modulated by descending pathways from the cortex, the hypothalamus and some brainstem nuclei in the brainstem [15] participating in perception and modulation of nociceptive sensation. Of these, especially important to note is the raphe magnus that has been shown to show changes in migraine implicating this area as the prime modifier of excitatory firing and that modulates serotonin secretion, a neurochemical that is heavily implicated in migraine pathogenesis and levels are low in migraine [35, 36]. The periaqueductal grey region is another area responsible for modulation of nociceptive sensation of the MSTN [35] that connects to the fourth ventricle constituting the vestibular nuclei. Therefore, it can be seen that classical migraine pathways and VM pathways merge centrally, thereby suggesting a common origin of symptoms.

The classical vascular theory as discussed above cannot be backed up by objective evidence; however, it is clear that vascular dynamics is affected during migraine. Vasoactive peptides given earlier include CGRP, neurokines and substance P that are secreted as a result of nociceptive receptor activation in the perivascular meninges by the migrainous excitatory firing. The resultant vascular changes initiate a secondary inflammatory response by mast cell degranulation and plasma cell extravasation with inflammatory substrates [33, 35]. This is called neurogenic inflammation that sensitises first-, second- and third-order neurones of the TVS. This sensitisation results in heightened response to both non-nociceptive and nociceptive stimuli and emergence of spontaneous activity [34]. This explains all of migraine's classical phenotypes.

2.3.3 Cortical Spreading Depression

It is still unclear as to how the initial migraine trigger is activated or initiated that leads to nociceptive meningeal receptor activation. One accepted theory is cortical spreading depression (CSD). This is characterised by neural depolarisation spreading from the occipital cortex and spreading towards the cortex followed by cortical suppression. This is mediated by an increase in intracellular calcium and extracellular Na+, K+, glutamate, NO and arachidonic acid in the synapses. This is an essentially excitatory wave that triggers the neurogenic inflammatory process in the TVS, leading to activation of the meningeal nociceptive receptors [37]. This explains the migraine aura but does not explain other symptoms. These other symptoms, e.g. the headache and the autonomic symptoms are attributed to a pathologically altered brain state where hyperexcitability of the TVS generates these symptoms [38]. It can be said that there is a fundamental sensory excitability or dysmodulation in migraine that leads to involve multiple sensations [39], which of course includes the vestibular sensation. This dysregulation may explain the different somatic sensations experienced in VM, e.g. photophobia, phonophobia, motion intolerance and sensory overload symptoms. The cause as to why some subjects are vulnerable to the migrainous process is unknown. Aetiological factor like genetics has been suggested. Secondary causes and associations of VM in, e.g. trauma or Meniere's disease (MD) will be discussed later.

The abovementioned has been researched in adults with functional studies, but there has been no study in the paediatric population. There are a few indirect pointers that a similar process activates the TVS in children suggested by overlapping of symptoms of VM with other conditions, e.g. epilepsy and juvenile head trauma syndrome, which follows milder form of head injuries in children [40]. There is a higher risk in epileptic children also sustaining migraine [41] although in the author's personal series of hundreds of paediatric VM, only a handful also suffered from epilepsy. This is discussed later. A lower ratio of cerebrospinal fluid to brain volume coupled with the developing cerebral plasticity driven by an evolving synaptic neuronal circuitry may be responsible to make a child's TVS more prone to migraine processes [42].

Table 2.1 shows the theories of pathogenesis of migraine.

2.3.4 Vestibular Substrates in VM

So far, we have discussed the genesis of the general migraine process. Now, we shall look and understand how the vestibular system might be affected in this process generating VM. Already we had a brief introduction that the TVS that is accepted as

Table 2.1 Theories of pathogenesis of migraine

Vascular
Trigeminovascular system activation
Cortical spreading depression
Inherent hyperexcitability, probably genetic

the key pathological pathway for migraine by its activation by CSD or de novo has connections to the vestibular nuclei through the periaqueductal grey zone.

VM differs from classical brainstem migraine as the key symptom of headache in the latter is replaced by dizziness/vertigo in the former. Dizziness/vertigo is a typical peripheral and/or central vestibular disorder, so it is rational to consider that the aforementioned TVS circuitry and its excitation predominantly involves the vestibular system and then spreads or simultaneously activates other components as in classical migraine.

The inner ear receives innervation from the ophthalmic branch of the trigeminal nerve through the basilar artery and the AICA [43] that in turn gives rise to the end artery vestibulocochlear artery. A release of neurotransmitters implicated in CSD as a result of TVS activation is also observed in the peripheral labyrinth by way of the same innervation that typifies TVS innervation of cranial blood vessels including the above. It has been also shown that activation of the TVS leads to a hyperdynamic circulation in the peripheral labyrinth and increased vascular permeability [33] that is typical of a neurogenic inflammation described above. This secondary inflammation may explain a nystagmus of peripheral origin found in VM. Interestingly, serotonin that plays a crucial role in classical migraine and that contributes to the neurogenic inflammatory response has also been detected in inner ear of rats [44].

Whilst it is tempting to suggest a peripheral vestibular pathology to explain the connecting link between VM and classical migraine, central mediators and pathways are equally important to consider. The most important caveat is that VM is because of reciprocal connections between nociceptive pathways triggered by the TVS circuitry and the vestibular processing areas in the brainstem. The vestibular processing areas in the brain are richly endowed with vast networking connections and include the vestibular nuclei, the parabrachial nuclei, the raphe nucleus and the locus coreleus [45]. The nociceptive TVS pathways not only generate the headache as seen earlier but also generate a vestibular counterpart in the form of dizziness/vertigo. The raphe nucleus plays a rather important role in modulating the central responses of VM.

The central vestibular pathways that merge with the TVS can be conceptualised in three parts: [46] firstly, a cognitive behavioural part involving the vestibulo-thalamo-cortical networks for final perception of vestibular, visual, proprioceptive and somatosensory afferents. Secondly, a sensorimotor component that with other brainstem nuclei regulates vestibular somatic, visceral and autonomic reflexes. Thirdly, an interoceptive component that translates vestibular information to subjective perceptions via the parabrachial nucleus, central amygdaloid nucleus, red nucleus of the stria terminalis, several posterior thalamic intralaminar nuclei, the hypothalamus and the insular cortex [46]. It is therefore not unsurprising that a migraine trigger activating the TVS by virtue of its overlapping vestibular connections also triggers a central vestibular phenotype. In this author's experience, several central oculomotor eye movements can occur in VM in children [47]. This is also common in adults [48].

Table 2.2 Vestibular areas participating in VM

Area	Location
Peripheral labyrinth supplied by vestibulocochlear artery	Inner ear
Uvula-nodulus, flocculus and the paraflocculus	Cerebellum
Vestibular nuclei	Brainstem
Raphe nucleus	Brainstem
Parabrachial nucleus	Brainstem
Locus coeruleus	Brainstem
Red nucleus	Midbrain
Thalamus	Diencephalon
Hypothalamus	Diencephalon
Amygdala	Temporal lobe
Hippocampus	Temporal lobe
Caudate nucleus	Basal ganglia in forebrain
Insula	Temporoparietal junction
Parietoinsular vestibular cortex	Parietal lobe

The vestibulo-cerebellar pathways incorporating the cerebellum are also activated in VM [49]. The uvula-nodulus, flocculus and the paraflocculus areas influence the vestibular system mostly by virtue of their rich connections to the vestibular nuclei [50] and functional imaging has indicated heightened activities during a VM. The hippocampus, amygdala, caudate nucleus, the hypothalamus, the insula, the parabrachial nuclei and indeed other limbic system areas receive afferents from the vestibular nuclei and the main vestibular processing cortex at the parainsular vestibular cortex (PIVC) that are responsible for the subjective perception and the emotional reaction to VM [51, 52]. In this author's series (unpublished), there were two teenagers with aqueduct of Sylvius stenosis and heterotrophic calcification in the parathird ventricular region, who had a disproportionately severe emotional reaction to a vestibular migraine.

Table 2.2 summarises the different areas of peripheral and central vestibular participation in VM.

2.3.5 Cochlear Substrates in VM

The recently published Barany criteria for both adult and paediatric VM does not include cochlear and auditory symptoms as these symptoms make a concrete diagnosis of VM difficult. This is because,Meniere's disease (MD) and intralabyrinthine cochleovestibular anomalies generate a similar phenotype. The present author deems this to be a logical idea given the observation that auditory symptoms are not as common in VM than vestibular symptoms in VM and are obligatory in the non-VM disorders with overlapping symptoms for diagnosis.

The prevalence of cochlear symptoms in VM from pooled data suggests a prevalence of about 12.2% [53] in adults and children combined. These include tinnitus, sensorineural hearing loss and aural fullness [54]. Otalgia is reported in 23% of school going children [55]. The hearing loss in most cases is reversible [53].

The relative dearth of cochlear symptoms in VM can be attributed to the observation that in contrast to the extensive connections of the TVS to the central vestibular afferent and efferent pathways, its connections to the central cochlear pathways are relatively less extensive. The TVS communicates with the dorsal cochlear nucleus and the superior colliculus [56]. The trigeminal ganglion innervates the cochlear blood vessels with the ophthalmic division; therefore, it does incorporate important peripheral and central cochlear pathways in the migraine circuitry. However, upstream modulation is still possible to dampen the auditory migraine circuitry as higher cochlear centres from beyond the superior colliculus (e.g. the olivary complex, the lateral lemniscus, medial geniculate body in the thalamus and the auditory cortex) are likely to be unaffected or less affected by TVS activation. In contrast, vestibular projections to the thalamus are widespread, including in the ventroposterior complex, the ventroanterior-ventrolateral complex, the intralaminar nuclei and the posterior nuclear group [57] that influence central inhibition of the TVS random firing in VM. Special mention must be made of the ventroposterior complex of the thalamus that receives direct connections from the trigeminal complex and the vestibular nuclei [32].

Figure 2.1 illustrates the pathogenesis of VM in children.

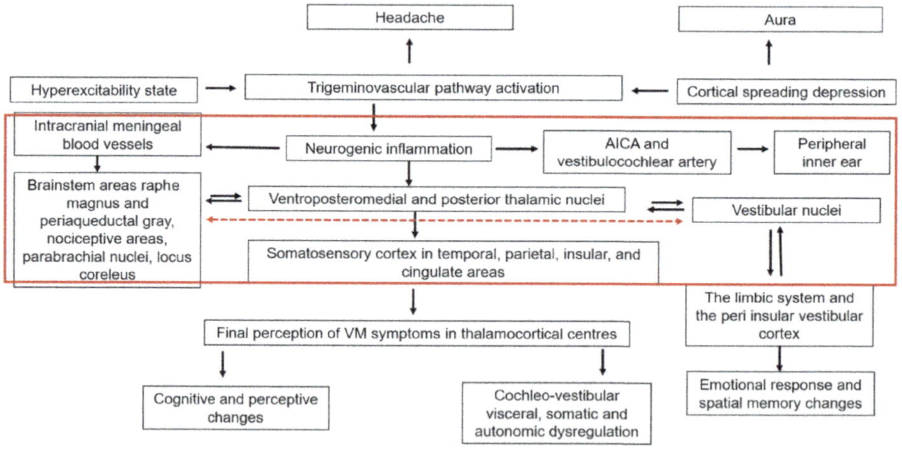

Fig. 2.1 Pathogenesis of VM in children. Red box shows merging of classical migraine and VM pathways. Limbic system—amygdala, hippocampus, posterior hypothalamus, caudate nucleus, cingular and insular cortex. Nociceptive areas—amygdala, hypothalamus, periaqueductal grey, basal ganglia, dorsolateral pontine tegmentum, rostroventral medulla, insular and cingular cortex

2.4 Neuropeptides, Neurotransmitters, Biomolecules and Hormones Implicated in VM

We have already discussed the role of serotonin in the raphe nucleus with its vascular effects and a balance between glutamate and GABA as important chemical mediators in TVS activation. We have also seen that different neuropeptides, including NAA, tCho, taurine and glutamate, participate in cerebral plasticity in a developing child's brain. There are numerous neurochemicals that are implicated in the migraine vis-a-vis VM process, of which a few deserve special mention. Knowledge regarding these neuropeptides is essential as their understanding drives pharmacological management of VM with targeted antagonism/inhibition of stimulation and promotion of inhibition of TVS activation. Pharmacological intervention in paediatric VM is covered in a different chapter. The readers are recommended a comprehensive article by Ahsina et al. [58] comprising of the original team who discovered TVS theory of migraine where neuropeptides and their applied importance for pharmacological management of migraine are discussed.

2.4.1 Neuropeptides

The main neurochemical protein that has been established across numerous studies is the calcium gene related peptide (CGRP). CGRP is widely distributed across the whole trigeminal circuitry, including the TVS, and is a very potent vasodilator. It is likely that CGRP mediates the cerebral vasodilatation associated with TVS activation that is responsible for neurogenic inflammation and transmission of the TVS nociceptive signals to other parts of the brain [34]. In the paediatric population, again, there is limited evidence as to the role CGRP in migraineurs. A review article whilst observing some similarities with the adult population inferred that there is a CGRP dependant and a CGRP independent group among children with migraine [40]. Given that VM and classical migraine pathways merge above the vestibular nuclei in the brainstem, CGRP does appear to be an important mediator in paediatric VM.

Substance P and neurokinins are the second group of similar peptides heavily expressed in the TVS that contribute to the neurogenic inflammation found in migraine/VM. These peptides contribute to nociception, excitatory synaptic transmission and neuroimmunomodulation [59]. NMDA receptors regulate the secretion of SP and CGRP activates NMDA receptors [60]. NMDA is a primarily an excitatory glutamate receptor that leads to spiking activities seen in migraine. Serotonin-driven dopamine inhibition has been proposed to augment migraine hypersenstivity [61] to a certain extent. DOPA receptors are observed in vestibular nuclei [62] in addition to their abundance in the thalamus and the basal ganglia.

A third protein pituitary adenylate cyclase-activating polypeptide (PACAP) has been proposed to influence the migraine process like the CGRP. Its receptors are also distributed along the TVS pathway, especially in the sphenopalatine ganglion and less in the trigeminal ganglion. It is a potent vasodilator as well and participates in the neurogenic inflammatory process [63]. It has not been studied as widely as the CGRP.

2.4.2 Neurotransmitters

It is known that migraine activity is partly due to imbalance between excitatory and inhibitory neurotransmission mediated by dedicated neurotransmitters glutamate and GABA and by a low secretion of serotonin. However, the specific neuroanatomical substrate that incorporates a specific neurotransmitter elaborated in a specific site of the vestibular-TVS common pathway remains elusive. A study by Zhang et al. [64] identified a glutamatergic projection from the trigeminal nucleus caudalis to the vestibular nuclei, which mediates vestibular dysfunction in the animal model. CGRP expressing neurones were connected to these glutaminergic neurones of the trigeminal nuclei. This connecting link does suggest that the vestibular nuclei are directly affected in the TVS migraine process.

2.4.3 Other Chemicals and Hormones

Nerve growth factor (NGF), nitric oxide, prostaglandins and capsaicin have all been implicated in influencing a migraine response by virtue of nociceptive modulation of the TVS [59]. These agents act on the neurogenic inflammatory response of VM.

The hormonal environment in perimenopausal women can be defined as unstable during the transition period of premenopausal to post menopause. The fluctuating ovarian hormones during this period are known to affect both glutamate and GABA receptor activity in the brain in addition to their serotonergic activity. As a result, they can trigger off a VM phenotype [65]. In post-menopausal women, estradiol levels were negatively correlated to VM intensity, duration and frequency [66]. The same hormonal fluctuations also lead to an increased and heightened propensity of acute migraine spells in menarche and pregnancy [67]. The effects of hormones have not been studied in VM in children.

The role of Vitamin B2 or Riboflavin has generated some interest when it was discovered that Vitamin B2 supplementation in a therapeutic dose is beneficial for any migraine including VM. The mechanism is likely to be at the level of mitochondrial oxidative phosphorylation for which Vitamin B2 is required [68]. Abnormalities of such mitochondrial action have been implicated in migraine [34].

Table 2.3 illustrates different chemicals involved in VM.

Table 2.3 Neuropeptides, neurotransmitters, biomolecules and hormones implicated in VM

Neuropeptides Calcitonin gene related peptide (CGRP) Substance P Neurokinin Pituitary adenylate cyclase-activating polypeptide (PACAP)	**Neurotransmitters** Glutamate Gamma-amino butyric acid (GABA) Serotonin Dopamine
Biomolecules Nerve growth factor (NGF) Nitric oxide Prostaglandins Capsaicin Riboflavin	**Hormones** Oestrogen Progesterone

2.5 Aetiology of VM in Children and Comorbid Pathologies

2.5.1 Genetic Factors

A genetic mutation leading to abnormalities in mitochondrial oxidative phosphorylation, channelopathy and magnesium homeostasis that is implicated in the migraine hyperexcitability and hypersensitisation state has been proposed, although not many genes have been definitely identified or replicated [34].

A familial history of migraine was observed in 70% of a population of VM, whereas 21.4% of VM sufferers had a positive familial history of migraine as found in a large metanalysis [69]. A review article scoping VM in children has observed that 75.6% of children with VM demonstrate a positive family history [70]. Genome-wide association studies so far have identified several consistent genes in migraineurs that include the PRDM16, TRPM8 and the LRP1 genes [35]. A large meta-analysis conducted in 2013 identified 12 definite and 134 probable loci for migraine suscpetibility [71]. Genetic VM appears to be polygenic.

The CACNA1 1 A gene that plays an important role in calcium homeostasis including in calcium ion gated channels when mutates generates three conditions: spinocerebellar ataxia type 2, episodic ataxia type 6 and familial hemiplegic migraine [35], and it is the only gene that has been definitely identified to cause some form of migraine. Since calcium as an ion is pivotal for extracellular signalling in the brain, it is likely that a calcium channelopathy will lead to abnormal TVS activity necessary for migraine excitability. Other probable loci discovered include a region in chromosome 11q and 5q.35 and in the genes ATP1A2, HTR6, PRG and TRPM7 in families with VM [44, 46, 69, 72].

2.5.2 Head Injury

VM after a head injury can be difficult to tease out from post-traumatic headache and dizziness. There had been no studies that have specifically studied VM after a head injury. Migrainous features appearing after a head trauma may occur in both children and in adults [40, 73]. The reported incidence in adults is 0.36% [74] and unknown in children. It is poorly correlated to the severity of the injury [75].

Various theories have been proposed to explain the development of migraine after a traumatic head injury. There is likely an elevation of extracellular potassium from such injuries leading to depolarisation and release of excitatory neurotransmitters [76], the head injury itself provoking neuroinflammation that is observed in migraine [74]. In children, CSD extension in head injuries is facilitated by CSF dynamics in a developing brain [40].

2.5.3 Epilepsy

William Gower in 1906 was the first to point out that epilepsy and migraine share several commonalities and that the latter often occur together [77]. Children with migraine has a 3.2–4.5 increased chance of developing an epilepsy [40, 78]. The hyperexcitability state that is a hallmark of both epilepsy and migraine is probably driven by genetic factors and/or secondary factors, e.g. a head injury [79]. Genetic mutations in CACNA1 1A and ATP1A2 can cause both migraine and focal seizures [79] and the observation that migraine and VM can both be treated by anti-epileptic drugs points out to a common pathophysiology.

The underlying mechanism is believed to lie in some form of channelopathy in both the conditions. The fundamental difference is that whilst in epilepsy, glutamate-driven AMPTA receptor is implicated for hyperexcitability, in migraine, the main excitatory substrate is the glutamate and CGRP-driven NMDA receptor in CSD [79]. There are fundamental differences in an epileptiform focus spread and CSD in terms of duration, velocity of spread and areas of spread. In epilepsy, the focus spreads more quickly and does not spread as broadly as the CSD [78]. Nevertheless, both the focal seizure and migraine including VM will eventually affect a cortical spread and merge at some point in the brainstem—thalamico-cortical pathways. So the phenotype of these two conditions although quite different share some common features, e.g. the autonomic symptoms involving sensory processes, headache and dizziness. The natural history is however different.

In children who are unable to provide a proper history or where parents/carers narrate a history observing their wards, it is not infrequently difficult to understand the so-called spells that a child might show. For example, both in VM and in epilepsy, the child may stop in their tracks, develop a vacant stare, shut their eyes and drop to the floor. Many of these children may receive a diagnosis of a focal epilepsy when they could have sustained VM. Therefore, according to the current author, given the lack of a robust and sensitive biomarker for VM, Barany's fourth criteria, i.e. exclusion of other causes is the most important diagnostic marker. Biomarkers for epilepsy like EEG and imaging findings are additional clues to a diagnosis of an epilepsy rather than VM.

2.5.4 Meniere's Disease (MD)

In adults, the comorbidity of MD and VM is well known [80]. In fact, patients with MD have a twofold risk of developing VM and MD and VM coexist together in at least 25% of subjects [81]. Diagnosis may be difficult due to overlapping symptoms and the common episodic dizziness phenotype. The Barany criteria for MD and VM are different [82]. Briefly, whilst MD is primarily a cochleovestibular disorder where hearing loss/aural fullness is an essential criterion for diagnosis, in VM, it is a primarily vestibular disorder where photophobia/phonophobia are essential criteria for diagnosis. However, by no means are aural symptoms exclusive to MD and autonomic features exclusive to VM.

Accepted MD and VM pathogenesis, i.e. endolymphatic hydrops and TVS hyperexcitability are not similar, so it is still not clear as to why there two conditions share phenotypes. The only common ground for pathogenesis is the underperfusion of the cochleovestibular artery that occurs in both to a certain extent. Why does this ischaemia selectively affect the cochlear territory in MD and the vestibular territory in VM is unknown.

Primary idiopathic MD is rare in children [83]. Overall MD prevalence in children is 2.3% [84]. It is usually secondary following autoimmune conditions or head injury [83]. The duration of episodic spells with dizziness is different in VM and MD and vestibular function tests can distinguish between the two in some instances. Chronic MD is more liable to generate vestibular weakness than VM. Cognitive and psychological effects are more pronounced in VM in children, not unsurprisingly because VM is a primarily central disorder unlike MD that is peripheral.

2.5.5 Classical Migraine

It can be noted that one of the criteria for diagnosis of VM in children is that 50% of the episodes have to be accompanied with a migrainous headache and there needs to be a history of migraine with or without aura. This inherently suggests that VM in children for a concrete diagnosis requires classical migraine to be present. This is a simplistic approach and frequently a classical migraine history is not obtained making the presentation far more complex that is not helped by a lack of anamnesis. Much more frequent is the observation that children rather fit the diagnosis of a probable VM where either a simultaneous history of a migraine is present or at least one migraine feature is present in addition to the dizziness, i.e. either headache or photophobia or phonophobia. A review indicated that up to 70% of children with VM may present with headache but by no means it is observed in all children [85].

Therefore, the association of VM and classical migraine in children is tenuous. Studies exploring the association in adults are also variable. Strict diagnostic criteria may lead to selection bias where the distinction between a VM and a classical migraine presenting with vertigo becomes blurred. There could be instances where criteria might not be fulfilled, yet, the child in question has a severely debilitating life style with vertigo. As emphasised earlier, diagnosis of VM in children is highly complex and a carefully weighted judgement is essential. It is wise to consider that VM and migrainous headache with vertigo belong to the same group of a hyperexcitable episodic central disorders and treated similarly [86].

2.5.6 Neurodevelopmental Disorders

We have already seen that autism and attention disorders increase the risk of migraine in children [20]. This is because of the balance between glutamate excitation and inhibition is tipped towards the excitation side in both autism and VM. Furthermore, it has been observed that autistic children are low on serotonin that also plays a critical role in VM and any migraine is essentially a 'low serotonin syndrome' [87]. All of these conditions present with sensory dysregulation mediated by common central pathways in the thalamocortical territory [88].

There is a lack of studies that have investigated the relative prevalence of migraine in autistic children. One study incorporating over 18,000 children observed that children with autism have a 2.75 times increased risk of developing migraine than non-autistic children [89]. Children who are autistic and who are also showing features of migraine have increased or heightened sensory dysregulation symptoms than autistic children without migraine [90].

The issue of attention disorders and migraine in children similarly has seen limited investigation. One study incorporating 81,000 children observed a 1.92 times increased risk of migraine in children with ADHD as compared to children without ADHD [91].

Diagnosing VM in children with neurodevelopmental disorders is a significant challenge as some symptoms merge and may be difficult to be noticed by the parents or the carers. Indirect surrogate history is determined by leading questions to describe vestibular behaviour that can sometimes be trivial or innocuous. However, it is possible with experience and the art of diagnosis.

Table 2.4 shows the associations of paediatric VM.

Table 2.4 Aetiology and comorbidities with VM

1. Classical migraine
2. Genetic factors—CACNA1 1A, ATP1A2, HTR6, PRG and TRPM7, chromosome 11q and 5q.35
3. Head injury
4. Epilepsy
5. Meniere's disease
6. Neurodevelopmental disorders

References

1. https://ichd-3.org/1-migraine/. 2024. Accessed 06.06.2024 at 8.15 AM.
2. Rose FC. The history of migraine from Mesopotamian to medieval times. Cephalalgia. 1995;15(Suppl 15):1–3. https://doi.org/10.1111/J.1468-2982.1995.
3. Liveing E. On megrim, sick-headache, and some allied disorders: a contribution to the pathology of nerve-storms. London: Churchill; 1873. p. 120–30.
4. Bickerstaff ER. Basilar artery migraine. Lancet. 1961;i:15–7.
5. Kayan A, Hood JD. Neuro-otological manifestations of migraine. Brain. 1984;107(Pt 4):1123–42. https://doi.org/10.1093/brain/107.4.1123.
6. Neuhauser H, Lempert T. Vertigo and dizziness related to migraine: a diagnostic challenge. Cephalalgia. 2004;24(2):83–91. https://doi.org/10.1111/j.1468-2982.2004.00662.x.
7. Lempert T, Olesen J, Furman J, Waterston J, Seemungal B, Carey J, Bisdorff A, Versino M, Evers S, Kheradmand A, Newman-Toker D. Vestibular migraine: diagnostic criteria1. J Vestib Res. 2022;32(1):1–6. https://doi.org/10.3233/VES-201644.
8. Basser LS. Benign paroxysmal vertigo of childhood: a variety of vestibular neuronitis. Brain. 1964;87:141–52.
9. Fenichel GM. Migraine as a cause of benign paroxysmal vertigo of childhood. J Pediatr. 1967;71:114–5.
10. Batson G. Benign paroxysmal vertigo of childhood: a review of the literature. Paediatr Child Health. 2004;9(1):31–4. https://doi.org/10.1093/pch/9.1.31.
11. van de Berg R, Widdershoven J, Bisdorff A, Evers S, Wiener-Vacher S, Cushing SL, Mack KJ, Kim JS, Jahn K, Strupp M, Lempert T. Vestibular migraine of childhood and recurrent vertigo of childhood: diagnostic criteria consensus document of the Committee for the Classification of Vestibular Disorders of the Bárány Society and the International Headache Society. J Vestib Res. 2021;31(1):1–9. https://doi.org/10.3233/VES-200003.
12. Wiener-Vacher SR, Quarez J, Priol AL. Epidemiology of vestibular impairments in a pediatric population. Semin Hear. 2018;39(3):229–42. https://doi.org/10.1055/s-0038-1666815.
13. O'Reilly RC, et al. Comprehensive vestibular and balance testing in the dizzy pediatric population. Otolaryngol Head Neck Surg. 2011;144(2):142–8. https://doi.org/10.1177/0194599810393679.
14. Dasgupta S, Mandala M, Salerni L, et al. Dizziness and balance problems in children. Curr Treat Options Neurol. 2020;22:8. https://doi.org/10.1007/s11940-020-0615-9.
15. Huang T-C, Wang S-J, Kheradmand A. Vestibular migraine: an update on current understanding and future directions. Cephalalgia. 2020;40(1):107–21. https://doi.org/10.1177/0333102419869317.
16. Perdue MV, DeMayo MM, Bell TK, Boudes E, Bagshawe M, Harris AD, Lebel C. Changes in brain metabolite levels across childhood. NeuroImage. 2023;274:120087. https://doi.org/10.1016/j.neuroimage.2023.120087.
17. de Tommaso M, Ceci E, Pica C, Trojano M, Delussi M, Franco G, Livrea P, Ruggieri M. Serum levels of N-acetyl-aspartate in migraine and tension-type headache. J Headache Pain. 2012;13(5):389–94. https://doi.org/10.1007/s10194-012-0448-3.
18. Zhang L, Huang J, Zhang Z, Cao Z. Altered metabolites in the occipital lobe in migraine without Aura during the attack and the Interictal period. Front Neurol. 2021;12:656349. https://doi.org/10.3389/fneur.2021.656349.
19. Martami F, Holton KF. Targeting glutamate neurotoxicity through dietary manipulation: potential treatment for migraine. Nutrients. 2023;15(18):3952. https://doi.org/10.3390/nu15183952.
20. Rubenstein JLR. Three hypotheses for developmental defects that may underlie some forms of autism spectrum disorder. Curr Opin Neurol. 2010;23(2):118–23. https://doi.org/10.1097/WCO.0B013E328336EB13.

21. Blüml S, Wisnowski JL, Nelson MD Jr, Paquette L, Gilles FH, Kinney HC, Panigrahy A. Metabolic maturation of the human brain from birth through adolescence: insights from in vivo magnetic resonance spectroscopy. Cereb Cortex. 2013;23(12):2944–55. https://doi.org/10.1093/cercor/bhs283.
22. Martínez F, Castillo J, Leira R, Prieto JM, Lema M, Noya M. Taurine levels in plasma and cerebrospinal fluid in migraine patients. Headache. 1993;33(6):324–7. https://doi.org/10.1111/j.1526-4610.1993.hed3306324.x.
23. Takahashi T, Shirane R, Sato S, Yoshimoto T. Developmental changes of cerebral blood flow and oxygen metabolism in children. AJNR Am J Neuroradiol. 1999;20(5):917–22.
24. Youssef PE, Mack KJ. Episodic and chronic migraine in children. Dev Med Child Neurol. 2020;62:34–41.
25. Johnston MV, Ishida A, Ishida WN, Matsushita HB, Nishimura A, Tsuji M. Plasticity and injury in the developing brain. Brain and Development. 2009;31(1):1–10. https://doi.org/10.1016/j.braindev.2008.03.014. Epub 2008
26. Lau CG, Zukin RS. NMDA receptor trafficking in synaptic plasticity and neuropsychiatric disorders. Nat Rev Neurosci. 2007;8(6):413–26.
27. Baloh RW. Neurotology of migraine. Headache. 1997;37:615–21. https://doi.org/10.1097/WCO.0b013e32836085f4.
28. Lee H. Isolated vascular vertigo. J Stroke. 2014;16:124–30. https://doi.org/10.5853/jos.2014.16.3.124.
29. May A, Goadsby PJ. The trigeminovascular system in humans: pathophysiologic implications for primary headache syndromes of the neural influences on the cerebral circulation. J Cereb Blood Flow Metab. 1999;19(2):115–27. https://doi.org/10.1097/00004647-199902000-00001.
30. Qubty W, Patniyot I. Migraine pathophysiology. Pediatr Neurol. 2020;107:1–6. https://doi.org/10.1016/j.pediatrneurol.2019.12.014.
31. Pietrobon D, Moskowitz MA. Pathophysiology of migraine. Annu Rev Physiol. 2013;75:365–91.
32. Price S, Daly DT. Neuroanatomy, trigeminal nucleus. 2023 May 1. In: StatPearls [Internet]. Treasure Island (FL): StatPearls Publishing; 2024.
33. Goadsby PJ, Charbit AR, Andreou AP, Akerman S, Holland PR. Neurobiology of migraine. Neuroscience. 2009;161(2):327–41. https://doi.org/10.1016/j.neuroscience.2009.03.019.
34. Ruthirago D, Julayanont P, Kim J. Chapter 7.2—Translational correlation: migraine. In: Conn PM, editor. Conn's translational neuroscience. Academic Press; 2017. p. 159–65. https://doi.org/10.1016/B978-0-12-802381-5.00013-0.
35. Espinosa-Sanchez JM, Lopez-Escamez JA. New insights into pathophysiology of vestibular migraine. Front Neurol. 2015;6:12. https://doi.org/10.3389/fneur.2015.00012.
36. Deen M, Hansen HD, Hougaard A, Nørgaard M, Eiberg H, Lehel S, Ashina M, Knudsen GM. High brain serotonin levels in migraine between attacks: a 5-HT4 receptor binding PET study. Neuroimage Clin. 2018;18:97–102. https://doi.org/10.1016/j.nicl.2018.01.016.
37. Zhang X, Levy D, Noseda R, Kainz V, Jakubowski M, Burstein R. Activation of meningeal nociceptors by cortical spreading depression: implications for migraine with aura. J Neurosci. 2010;30:8807–14. https://doi.org/10.1523/JNEUROSCI.0511-10.2010.
38. Charles A. Migraine: a brain state. Curr Opin Neurol. 2013;26:235–9. https://doi.org/10.1097/WCO.0b013e32836085f4.
39. Goadsby PJ, Holland PR, Martins-Oliveira M, et al. Pathophysiology of migraine: a disorder of sensory processing. Physiol Rev. 2017;97:553–622.
40. Førland-Schill A, Berring-Uldum A, Debes NM. Migraine pathophysiology in children and adolescents: a review of the literature. J Child Neurol. 2022;37(7):642–51. https://doi.org/10.1177/08830738221100888.
41. Rajapakse T, Buchhalter J. The borderland of migraine and epilepsy in children. Headache. 2016;56(6):1071–80. https://doi.org/10.1111/head.12827.

42. Moskowitz M, Nozaki K, Kraig R. Neocortical spreading depression provokes the expression of c-fos protein-like immunoreactivity within trigeminal nucleus caudalis via trigeminovascular mechanisms. J Neurosci. 1993;13(3):1167–77. https://doi.org/10.1523/JNEUROSCI.13-03-01167.1993.
43. Vass Z, Shore SE, Nuttall AL, Miller JM. Direct evidence of trigeminal innervation of the cochlear blood vessels. Neuroscience. 1998;84:559–67. https://doi.org/10.1016/S0306-4522(97)00503-4.
44. Sohn JH. Recent advances in the understanding of vestibular migraine. Behav Neurol. 2016;2016:1801845. https://doi.org/10.1155/2016/1801845.
45. Balaban CDL. Anterograde tracing of projections from the dorsal raphe nucleus to the vestibular nuclei. Neuroscience. 2006;143:641–54. https://doi.org/10.1016/j.neuroscience.2006.08.013.
46. Furman JM, Marcus DA, Balaban CD. Vestibular migraine: clinical aspects and pathophysiology. Lancet Neurol. 2013;12(7):706–15. https://doi.org/10.1016/S1474-4422(13)70107-8.
47. Crunkhorn R, Ratnayake S. Dasgupta S1747 Vestibular Migraine in Children. Arch Dis Child. 2021;106:A475.
48. Dieterich M, Brandt T. Episodic vertigo related to migraine (90 cases): vestibular migraine? J Neurol. 1999;246:883–92.
49. Li P, Gu H, Xu J, Zhang Z, Li F, Feng M, Tian Q, Shang C, Zhuang J. Purkinje cells of vestibulocerebellum play an important role in acute vestibular migraine. J Integr Neurosci. 2019;18(4):409–14. https://doi.org/10.31083/j.jin.2019.04.1168.
50. Neal H. Barmack, Central vestibular system: vestibular nuclei and posterior cerebellum. Brain Res Bull. 2003;60(5–6):511–41. https://doi.org/10.1016/S0361-9230(03)00055-8.
51. Rajagopalan A, Jinu KV, Sailesh KS, Mishra S, Reddy UK, Mukkadan JK. Understanding the links between vestibular and limbic systems regulating emotions. J Nat Sci Biol Med. 2017;8(1):11–5. https://doi.org/10.4103/0976-9668.198350.
52. May A, Burstein R. Hypothalamic regulation of headache and migraine. Cephalalgia. 2019;39(13):1710–9. https://doi.org/10.1177/0333102419867280. Epub 2019 Aug 29
53. Hwang JH, Tsai SJ, Liu TC, Chen YC, Lai JT. Association of tinnitus and other cochlear disorders with a history of migraines. JAMA Otolaryngol Head Neck Surg. 2018;144(8):712–7. https://doi.org/10.1001/jamaoto.
54. Shi S, Wang D, Ren T, Wang W. Auditory manifestations of vestibular migraine. Front Neurol. 2022;13:944001. https://doi.org/10.3389/fneur.2022.944001.
55. Anttila P, Metsähonkala L, Mikkelsson M, Helenius H, Sillanpää M. Comorbidity of other pains in schoolchildren with migraine or nonmigrainous headache. J Pediatr. 2001;138(2):176–80. https://doi.org/10.1067/mpd.2001.112159.
56. Shore SE, Vass Z, Wys NL, Altschuler RA. Trigeminal ganglion innervates the auditory brainstem. J Comp Neurol. 2000;419(3):271–85. https://doi.org/10.1002/(sici)1096-9861(20000410)419:3<271::aid-cne1>3.0.co;2-m.
57. Wijesinghe R, Protti DA, Camp AJ. Vestibular interactions in the thalamus. Front Neural Circuits. 2015;9:79. https://doi.org/10.3389/fncir.2015.00079.
58. Ashina M, Hansen JM, Do TP, Melo-Carrillo A, Burstein R, Moskowitz MA. Migraine and the trigeminovascular system-40 years and counting. Lancet Neurol. 2019;18(8):795–804. https://doi.org/10.1016/S1474-4422(19)30185-1.
59. Malhotra R. Understanding migraine: potential role of neurogenic inflammation. Ann Indian Acad Neurol. 2016;19(2):175–82. https://doi.org/10.4103/0972-2327.182302.
60. Guerrero-Toro C, Koroleva K, Ermakova E, Gafurov O, Abushik P, Tavi P, Sitdikova G, Giniatullin R. Testing the role of glutamate NMDA receptors in peripheral trigeminal nociception implicated in migraine pain. Int J Mol Sci. 2022;23(3):1529. https://doi.org/10.3390/ijms23031529.
61. Mascia A, Afra J, Schoenen J. Dopamine and migraine: a review of pharmacological, biochemical, neurophysiological, and therapeutic data. Cephalalgia. 1998;18(4):174–82. https://doi.org/10.1046/j.1468-2982.1998.1804174.x.

62. Vibert N, Serafin M, Crambes O, Vidal PP, Mühlethaler M. Dopaminergic agonists have both presynaptic and postsynaptic effects on the Guinea-pig's medial vestibular nucleus neurons. Eur J Neurosci. 1995;7(4):555–62. https://doi.org/10.1111/j.1460-9568.1995.tb00660.x.
63. Kuburas A, Russo AF. Shared and independent roles of CGRP and PACAP in migraine pathophysiology. J Headache Pain. 2023;24:34. https://doi.org/10.1186/s10194-023-01569-2.
64. Zhang Y, Zhang Y, Wang Y, Zhang X, Qin G, Zhang D, Chen L, Zhou J. Inhibition of glutamatergic trigeminal nucleus caudalis-vestibular nucleus projection neurons attenuates vestibular dysfunction in the chronic-NTG model of migraine. J Headache Pain. 2023;24(1):77. https://doi.org/10.1186/s10194-023-01607-z.
65. Park JH, Viirre E. Vestibular migraine may be an important cause of dizziness/vertigo in perimenopausal period. Med Hypotheses. 2010;75(5):409–14. https://doi.org/10.1016/j.mehy.2009.04.054.
66. Tang B, Yu X, Jiang W, Zhang C, Zhan T, He Y. Clinical significance of serum sex hormones in postmenopausal women with vestibular migraine: potential role of estradiol. J Int Med Res. 2021;49(5):3000605211016379. https://doi.org/10.1177/03000605211016379.
67. Sacco S, Ricci S, Degan D, Carolei A. Migraine in women: the role of hormones and their impact on vascular diseases. J Headache Pain. 2012;13(3):177–89. https://doi.org/10.1007/s10194-012-0424-y.
68. Chen YS, Lee HF, Tsai CH, Hsu YY, Fang CJ, Chen CJ, et al. Effect of vitamin B2 supplementation on migraine prophylaxis: a systematic review and meta-analysis. Nutr Neurosci. 2021;25(9):1801–12. https://doi.org/10.1080/1028415X.2021.1904542.
69. Paz-Tamayo A, Perez-Carpena P, Lopez-Escamez JA. Systematic review of prevalence studies and familial aggregation in vestibular migraine. Front Genet. 2020;11:954. https://doi.org/10.3389/fgene.2020.00954.
70. Saniasiaya J, Salim R. Characteristics and diagnostic approach of vestibular migraine in children and adolescents: a systematic review. Auris Nasus Larynx. 2023;50(2):218–27. https://doi.org/10.1016/j.anl.2022.06.007.
71. Anttila V, Winsvold BS, Gormley P, et al. Genome-wide meta-analysis identifies new susceptibility loci for migraine. Nat Genet. 2013;45(8):912–7. https://doi.org/10.1038/ng.2676.
72. Ceriani CEJ. Vestibular migraine pathophysiology and treatment: a narrative review. Curr Pain Headache Rep. 2024;28(2):47–54. https://doi.org/10.1007/s11916-023-01182-7.
73. Chen MH, Sung YF, Chien WC, Chung CH, Chen JW. Risk of migraine after traumatic brain injury and effects of injury management levels and treatment modalities: a nationwide population-based cohort study in Taiwan. J Clin Med. 2023;12(4):1530. https://doi.org/10.3390/jcm12041530.
74. Misale P, Hassannia F, Dabiri S, Brandstaetter T, Rutka J. Post-traumatic peripheral vestibular disorders (excluding positional vertigo) in workers following head injury. Sci Rep. 2021;11(1):23436. https://doi.org/10.1038/s41598-021-02987-5.
75. Packard RC, Ham LP. Pathogenesis of posttraumatic headache and migraine: a common headache pathway? Headache. 1997;37:142–52. https://doi.org/10.1046/j.1526-4610.1997.3703142.x.
76. Ruff RL, Blake K. Pathophysiological links between traumatic brain injury and post-traumatic headaches. F1000Research. 2016;5:1–11. https://doi.org/10.12688/f1000research.9017.1.
77. Gowers WR. Clinical lectures on the borderland of epilepsy. III.—migraine. Brit Med J. 1906;2(2397):1617–22.
78. Ludvigsson P, Hesdorffer D, Olafsson E, Kjartansson O, Hauser WA. Migraine with aura is a risk factor for unprovoked seizures in children. Ann Neurol. 2006;59:210–3.
79. Rogawski MA. Migraine and epilepsy—shared mechanisms within the family of episodic disorders. In: Noebels JL, Avoli M, Rogawski MA, et al., editors. Jasper's basic mechanisms of the epilepsies [internet]. 4th ed. Bethesda, MD: National Center for Biotechnology Information (US); 2012. https://www.ncbi.nlm.nih.gov/books/NBK98193/.
80. Radtke A, Lempert T, Gresty MA, et al. Migraine and Ménière's disease: is there a link? Neurology. 2002;59:1700–4. https://doi.org/10.1212/01.wnl.0000036903.22461.39.

81. Neff BA, Staab JP, Eggers SD, Carlson ML, Schmitt WR, Van Abel KM, Worthington DK, Beatty CW, Driscoll CL, Shepard NT. Auditory and vestibular symptoms and chronic subjective dizziness in patients with Ménière's disease, vestibular migraine, and Ménière's disease with concomitant vestibular migraine. Otol Neurotol. 2012;33(7):1235–44. https://doi.org/10.1097/MAO.0b013e31825d644a.
82. Lopez-Escamez JA, Carey J, Chung W-H, et al. Diagnostic criteria for Menière's disease. J Vestib Res. 2015;25(1):1–7. https://doi.org/10.3233/VES-150549.
83. Lopez-Escamez JA, Liu Y. Epidemiology and genetics of Menière's disease. Curr Opin Neurol. 2023; https://doi.org/10.1097/WCO.0000000000001227.
84. Brantberg K, Duan M, Falahat B. Ménière's disease in children aged 4-7 years. Acta Otolaryngol. 2012;132(5):505–9. https://doi.org/10.3109/00016489.2011.643240.
85. Langhagen T, Landgraf MN, Huppert D, et al. Vestibular migraine in children and adolescents. Curr Pain Headache Rep. 2016;20:67. https://doi.org/10.1007/s11916-016-0600-x.
86. Abouzari M, Goshtasbi K, Moshtaghi O, Tan D, Lin HW, Djalilian HR. Association between vestibular migraine and migraine headache: yet to explore. Otol Neurotol. 2020;41(3):392–6. https://doi.org/10.1097/MAO.0000000000002528.
87. Chugani DC, Muzik O, Behen M, Rothermel R, Janisse JJ, Lee J, Chugani HT. Developmental changes in brain serotonin synthesis capacity in autistic and nonautistic children. Ann Neurol. 1999;45:287–95. https://doi.org/10.1002/1531-8249(199903)45:3<287::AID-ANA3>3.0.CO;2-9.
88. Vetri L. Autism and migraine: an unexplored association? Brain Sci. 2020;10(9):615. https://doi.org/10.3390/brainsci10090615.
89. Lee T-Y, Tsai S-J, Chen T-J, Chen M-H. Risk of migraine development among children and adolescents with autism spectrum disorder: a nationwide longitudinal study. Res Autism Spectr Disord. 2021;89:101880. https://doi.org/10.1016/j.rasd.2021.101880.
90. Sullivan JC, Miller LJ, Nielsen DM, Schoen SA. The presence of migraines and its association with sensory hyperreactivity and anxiety symptomatology in children with autism spectrum disorder. Autism. 2014;18(6):743–7. https://doi.org/10.1177/1362361313489377.
91. Hsu TW, Chen MH, Chu CS, Tsai SJ, Bai YM, Su TP, Chen TJ, Liang CS. Attention deficit hyperactivity disorder and risk of migraine: a nationwide longitudinal study. Headache. 2022;62(5):634–41. https://doi.org/10.1111/head.14306.

Diagnosis and Relevant Investigations of Vestibular Migraine

3

Josine Widdershoven

3.1 Introduction

In order to comprehend the diagnostic process and relevant investigations in children and adolescents with symptoms of vestibular migraine, it is important understand the physiologic basis of the vestibular system.

3.2 Fundamental Basis of Physiology of Balance

When vestibular hair cells are stimulated by rotation, translation, or change in orientation in relation to gravity, the firing rate of the eighth nerve fibre innervating the corresponding hair cell increases or decreases. When the stereocilia bend towards the kinocilium, it depolarises the hair cell, increasing its firing rate in the eighth nerve fibre. In contrast, movements that bend the stereocilia away from the kinocilium decrease the neural firing in the eighth nerve. Besides the labyrinth, the vestibular nuclei receive information from other sensory systems, notably vision, somatic sensation, and hearing. Following the integration of sensory information, the output from vestibular nuclei influences eye movements, truncal stability, and spatial orientation.

The vestibular-ocular reflex is generated so the eye's visual axis stays on target during head movement. During the movement of the head, eye movement can be

J. Widdershoven (✉)
Department of Otorhinolaryngology, Maastricht University Medical Center, Maastricht, The Netherlands

Department of Otorhinolaryngology, Antwerp University Hospital, Antwerp, Belgium
e-mail: josine.widdershoven@mumc.nl

J. Saniasiaya (ed.), *Vestibular Migraine in Children and Adolescents: An overview*, https://doi.org/10.1007/978-981-96-2167-5_3

either equal to or opposite of the head movement, i.e., head movement to the left results in a rightward eye movement and vice versa. Additionally, for the horizontal system, the two vestibular nuclear complexes on each side of the brainstem work jointly so that when one nucleus is excited, the other is inhibited. The central nervous system (CNS) reciprocates the difference in the neural activity between the two vestibular complexes. In the instances when the head is static, the resting discharge is equal between the two vestibular nuclei. The CNS recognises the symmetrical neural activity, thus concluding that the head is static. However, during the head turn, for example, to the left, the endolymph flow results in an excitatory response to the side on which the head moves, which is the left, and simultaneously an inhibitory response on the opposite side, which is the right. Hence, the neural activity in both the vestibular nerve and nuclei, in this case, to the left and right, increases and decreases, respectively. The CNS detects the difference in neural activity between the two vestibular complexes as a head movement, resulting in vestibular-ocular and postural responses. This push–pull balance between the two labyrinths becomes affected following labyrinthine injury.

A sudden unilateral disruption of peripheral vestibular function leads to a loss of resting neural discharge activity of the corresponding vestibular nerve and nucleus. The CNS will detect the differences between the two labyrinths and interpret it as a rapid head movement towards the healthy labyrinth, resulting in vertigo. A "corrective" eye movement is generated to the opposite side, causing nystagmus, with the slow component towards the abnormal side and the fast component towards the healthy labyrinth [1].

3.3 Assessment of Children with Dizziness

During the first visit, a complete medical history, in addition to the chief presentation, should be gathered. This includes the comorbidities, associated complaints, family history, and medication history is essential.

Once history has been obtained, a thorough physical examination is carried out. Cranial nerve and ocular movement examination are included in this examination. Vestibular testing is performed if the diagnosis remains uncertain.

3.4 History

3.4.1 Chief Complaint

When obtaining the chief complaints, the child should describe the symptoms as they are perceived in his or her vocabulary. This should include the accompanying sensations, including nausea, vomiting, headache, and motion sickness. Relating the child's presentation to their own experience, such as riding a boat or carousel, will be useful. Nevertheless, it is imperative to gather information regarding the onset, duration, and frequency of dizziness as well as to relate the complaints or episodes of dizziness to specific activities. Reported factors that can trigger dizziness include alteration in position, coughing or sneezing, lack of sleep, as well as psychological strains.

The attending clinician should inquire about any associations with hearing loss, including its onset, progression, fluctuations, or improvement, the presence of tinnitus or aural fullness, and the laterality of these otologic complaints. Associated neurological manifestations, questions on seizure, altered behaviour or mental status, gait disturbances such as ataxia or weakness, presence of dysphagia, facial palsy, and visual disturbances should be gathered during the history taking.

3.5 Physical Examination

Apart from a thorough neurological examination, the clinician should observe the child when walking or running to look for any presence of any movement incoordination, such as ataxia.

Eye movement assessment, notably nystagmus, is vital when assessing a dizzy child. Spontaneous nystagmus is the presence of an involuntary, rhythmical movement of the eyes without external stimulation. It has two components: the slow component and the fast component. The fast component usually depicts the nystagmus. Spontaneous nystagmus can be elicited by asking the child to look straight ahead with and without fixation. In contrast, asking the child to look laterally with fixation (within 30 degrees) can assess the presence of gaze-evoked nystagmus. It is normal to find the presence of an end-gaze nystagmus when the eyes are completely deviated laterally.

Nystagmus or vertigo can be elicited through positional testing with specific manoeuvres. To elicit static position-related nystagmus, the child is placed in six different positions, including supine, sitting, and supine positions, with the head turned to the right and to the left, as well as right and left lateral positions. Position-related nystagmus is evoked the moment the child is placed in the position and can remain as long as the child is in the provoked position.

The vestibulospinal function is assessed using a foam pad either with or without a visual conflict dome.

Besides clinical anamnesis and clinical examination, vestibular testing is essential when evaluating a dizzy child. Vestibular testing is imperative when a complete history and examination fail to provide sufficient information to diagnose a child with dizziness. Vestibular testing can also aid in differentiating peripheral from central pathology, detect the site or laterality of the abnormality, and document the obtained finding, which can be useful to compare following intervention.

Vestibular tests that can be performed include vestibulocular and vestibulospinal tests, which can indirectly quantify the function of vestibular end organs.

3.6 Videonystagmography and Electronystagmography

Eye movements can be recorded using videonystagmography, a tool that uses infrared light which has been widely used worldwide. Dermal electrodes can also be easily applied in a child who is too young to wear video goggles for electronystagmography.

The common battery of vestibular testing, such as oculomotor tests, positional manoeuvres, and caloric tests, requires approximately 1 hour with discontinuation of certain medications, especially sedatives and vestibular suppressants, at least 2 days before the assessment.

The oculomotor test assesses neural motor output independent of the vestibular system. An abnormal finding in the oculomotor test can be misleading, resulting in a false positive result when the vestibular testing relies on eye movements. A computer-mediated sequence of target jumps can detect the saccade. The presence of a saccade can be classified into hypermetric saccades, or overshooting the target, and hypometric saccades, or undershooting the target. Typically, abnormality in the saccadic system is associated with CNS disorders.

To record spontaneous nystagmus and gaze-evoked nystagmus, the child is asked to look 30 degrees to each side, right and left, and the nystagmus can be recorded with and without fixation.

If the spontaneous nystagmus elicited in a dark room without fixation reduces or resolves during visual fixation, it is more suggestive of a peripheral vestibular condition. On the contrary, if the spontaneous nystagmus is present with fixation and is not reduced or improves with loss of fixation, it is most suggestive of a CNS abnormality.

To elicit smooth pursuit, the child is asked to follow a moving target along a slow, pendular path, back and forth. Typically, in a healthy child, the target can be followed smoothly without any interruption. Pursuit tracking abnormalities result from CNS lesions. On the other hand, when testing optokinetic nystagmus, black-and-white stripes moving to the left and right are used. Optokinetic nystagmus abnormalities, such as the presence of asymmetry and absence of response, indicate the presence of CNS lesions.

The positional test is conducted in static and dynamic conditions. Similar to the positional test performed during clinical examination, the child is placed in a sitting, supine, head, right–left turn, right, and left lateral position in a dark room. Typically, static positional nystagmus appears immediately as the child attains the provoked position and remains present as long as the child is in it.

Static positional nystagmus has been reported as a nonspecific and nonlocalising vestibular sign. The paroxysmal positional test includes the Dix–Hallpike manoeuvre, which revolves around positioning the child from a sitting position with the head straight, then turning the head 45 degrees to either the right or left side, and subsequently lying supine. At the same time, the head is still turned, and the neck extends 20°. The child is subsequently brought up to the sitting position, and the test is repeated on the opposite side.

The presence of nystagmus latency, rotational type of nystagmus, and attenuation is suggestive of benign paroxysmal positional vertigo (BPPV). Although BPPV is uncommon in children, its presence has been associated with a migraine variant.

3.7 Caloric Testing

The caloric test is able to individually assess each labyrinth by generating nystagmus following thermal stimulation of the vestibular system. The child will initially be placed supine with the head elevated 30° to make the horizontal semicircular canals lie in the vertical plane. The caloric stimulation will result in a convection current through the horizontal semicircular canal, which leads to a deflection of the cupula (into which the hairs of the hair cells are embedded) and a simultaneous change in the vestibular nerve activity. Cold irrigation results in a fast nystagmus beating away from the stimulated ear, while warm irrigation results in a fast nystagmus beating towards the stimulated ear. The common mnemonic *COWS*, "cold opposite, warm same," denotes the direction of the fast-beating nystagmus.

Binaural bi-thermal caloric testing utilises a stimulus of 30 and 44 °C, and each ear canal is irrigated for 30 s with 250 mL of water, with a 5-min rest period. Peak slow-component velocity of the nystagmus following the thermal stimulus has been identified as the most common method of measuring the caloric response that typically corresponds to the intensity of the vestibular response. Jongkees' formula is used to compare the responsiveness of one ear to the other ear, in order to compute a percentage of reduced vestibular response:

$$\left[\left[(\mathrm{R}30^\circ + \mathrm{R}44^\circ) - (\mathrm{L}30^\circ + \mathrm{L}44^\circ)\right] \Big/ \left[\mathrm{R}30^\circ + \mathrm{R}44^\circ + \mathrm{L}30^\circ + \mathrm{L}44^\circ\right]\right] \times 100 \text{ percent}$$

The normal limits have been reported when the vestibular response is reduced by more than 24%, whereby a reduced vestibular response indicates a peripheral vestibular lesion.

3.8 Rotational Testing

Rotation is a natural stimulus to the semicircular canals. The rotational test is typically well-tolerated, causing minimal discomfort to children, even infants and young children (who can be placed on a parent's lap). This test aims to stimulate the bilateral labyrinth concurrently, although it does not provide information regarding the side of the lesion. The caloric test and rotational test are typically complementary. The sinusoidal harmonic acceleration is the most common type of positional test. It is worth noting that the eye velocity formed by the rotation is comparable to the stimulus velocity.

From the rotational testing, three parameters can be obtained: gain, phase, and symmetry. Gain measures the size of the response, and when it is reduced, it indicates decreased vestibular sensitivity, typically bilateral vestibular loss. The gain obtained following a unilateral vestibular loss may or may not produce a reduced gain.

Phase indicates the relationship between rotational chair velocity and eye velocity timing. In an ideal eye movement, zero phase lead is obtained; on the contrary, large phase leads typically signify abnormality. Although a nonspecific measure of vestibular system abnormalities, phase has been found to be highly sensitive. The directional preponderance or the deviation from the symmetry of the eye movements is gathered by comparing the right and left velocities of the eye movement. Directional preponderance has been found to be a nonspecific sign. It is worth noting that gain, phase, and degree of symmetry do not indicate the laterality of the lesion. Yet, rotational tests can be used to monitor a child's progress as they measure the alteration in response to vestibular disease.

3.9 Computerised Dynamic Platform Posturography

Computerised dynamic posturography can assess a child's ability to use six different sensory conditions in individual or combinations of sensory inputs. The test uses a commercially developed machine, EquiTest® (NeuroCom International, Inc.), which comprises a floor and a moving visual scene.

For instance, Conditions 5 and 6 are evaluated by combining the floor and moving visual scene based on how the child responds to the vestibular input, as it is the only available sensory system providing reliable information. When the visual and somatosensory system is affected, the child is forced to depend on the vestibular system to maintain an upright balance.

It has been reported that following vestibular compensation, posturography results normalise, whereby children lose their "5,6 patterns," resulting in a normal postural sway [2]. Hence, posturography may provide important information regarding compensation status in a child with peripheral vestibular deficit.

3.10 Vestibular-Evoked Myogenic Potentials

Vestibular-evoked myogenic potentials (VEMPs) are obtained in response to intense auditory clicks through electrical activity recorded from the contracted neck muscles. VEMPs represent the status of otolith organs and their innervation: the sacculus, inferior vestibular nerve, and utricle and superior vestibular nerve.

If the test is performed using an air-conduction stimulus, a normal middle ear function is required to obtain a VEMP recording. Hence, in younger children who are typically prone to developing middle ear effusion, VEMP is conducted using a bone-conducted stimulus. VEMP has been successfully recorded in children as young as 3 months [3–5].

3.11 Video Head Impulse Test

Semicircular canal function can also be measured by determining the vestibular-ocular reflex (VOR) relative to head rotation. The VOR stabilises gaze by synchronously rotating the eyes in the opposite direction of the head movement. While the patient maintains gaze on a fixed target, the head is moved by sudden, small impulses in the plane of each pair of semicircular canals. When the patient is unable to maintain their focus on the fixed target after the onset of the head impulse, the eyes make a corrective saccade to return the gaze to the target (overt saccade) indicating a loss of VOR indicative of a peripheral vestibular loss. In the case of long term and/or congenital peripheral vestibular loss, the eyes are sometimes able to start the corrective saccade during the head impulse (covert saccade). Especially these covert saccades may be difficult to observe by the examiner while carrying out the test. For this reason, it is preferred to record the eye and head movements with a video system (video head impulse test, vHIT) with either video goggles or a standalone camera system (Wiener-Vacher, 2017; Gerdsen, 2024) [5, 6]. Though the vHIT is a convenient test in children, it does require a well-trained test administrator and (sometimes) a large number of impulses to obtain a reliable result. A possible solution has been proposed in the computerised rotational head impulse test (crHIT) (Mittendorff et al., 2023) [7].

3.12 Diagnosis of Vertigo in Children

Despite the multitude of possible vestibular tests mentioned above, most children have e diagnosis based on complaints and clinical criteria. However, the tests of vestibular function described above are important to rule out other disorders, such as unilateral or bilateral vestibular loss or CNS disorders.

3.13 Diagnostic Criteria of Vestibular Migraine of Childhood

Migraine is probably the most common cause of recurrent vertigo in children. Whereas migraine typically presents as headache in adults, other manifestations of migraine, including recurrent vertigo and disequilibrium, are more common in children. Unfortunately the prevalence of vestibular migraine in children remains unknown (Carmona et al. 2018) [8]. This is most likely caused by the fact that the majority of children with recurrent vertigo were previously diagnosed with benign paroxysmal vertigo of childhood as described by Basser in 1964 [9]. However, a number of these children also fit migraine criteria and develop migraine later in life. In order to separate these diagnoses in the International Classification of Vestibular Disorders distinct diagnostic criteria for vestibular migraine and recurrent vertigo of childhood have been proposed (van de Berg et al., 2021) [10].

The diagnostic criteria are as follows:

3.14 Vestibular Migraine of Childhood (VMC)

A. At least five episodes with vestibular symptoms of moderate or severe intensity lasting between 5 min and 72 h.
B. A current or past history of migraine with or without aura.
C. At least half of episodes are associated with at least one of the following three migraine features:

   1. Headache with at least two of the following four characteristics:

      (a) One-sided location.
      (b) Pulsating quality.
      (c) Moderate or severe pain intensity.
      (d) Aggravation by routine physical activity.

   2. Photophobia and phonophobia.
   3. Visual aura.

D. Age < 18 years.
E. Not better accounted for by another headache disorder, vestibular disorder, or other condition.

3.15 Probable Vestibular Migraine of Childhood (pVMC)

A. At least three episodes with vestibular symptoms of moderate or severe intensity lasting between 5 min and 72 h.
B. Only one of the criteria B and C for Vestibular Migraine of Childhood.
C. Age < 18 years.
D. Not better accounted for by another headache disorder, vestibular disorder, or other condition.

3.16 Recurrent Vertigo of Childhood (RVC)

In children who experience episodes of vertigo without migraine features the diagnosis of RVC should be considered. These episodes generally last only a few minutes and are not accompanied by loss of consciousness or other neurologic symptoms.

Recurrent Vertigo of Childhood (RVC)

A. At least three episodes with vestibular symptoms of moderate or severe intensity, lasting between 1 min and 72 h.
B. None of the criteria B and C for Vestibular Migraine of Childhood.
C. Age < 18 years.
D. Not better accounted for by another headache disorder, vestibular disorder, or other condition.

3.17 Differential Diagnosis

As mentioned earlier, it remains important to rule out other causes of vertigo in children, as evidenced in criteria D and E in the diagnostic criteria above. Van de Berg et al. have described other differential diagnoses elaborately, including Meniere's disease, episodic ataxia, posterior fossa tumours, and recurrent otitis media [10]. Additional testing, such as audiometry and/or radiologic examinations, may be needed to rule these out.

References

1. Swaiman Pediatric Neurology, 7th edition; to be published in 2025; chapter 8, authors Joe Furman and Josine Widdershoven.
2. Furman JM. Role of posturography in the management of vestibular patients. Otolaryngol Head Neck Surg. 1995;112(1):8–15.
3. Martens S, Dhooge I, Dhondt C, Vanaudenaerde S, Sucaet M, Van Hoecke H, De Leenheer E, Rombaut L, Boudewyns A, Desloovere C, Vinck AS, de Varebeke SJ, Verschueren D, Verstreken M, Foulon I, Staelens C, De Valck C, Calcoen R, Lemkens N, Öz O, De Bock M, Haverbeke L, Verhoye C, Declau F, Devroede B, Forton G, Deggouj N, Maes L. Three years of vestibular infant screening in infants with sensorineural hearing loss. Pediatrics. 2022;150:1.
4. Martens S, Dhooge I, Dhondt C, Vanaudenaerde S, Sucaet M, Rombaut L, Maes L. Pediatric vestibular assessment: clinical framework. Ear Hear. 2023;44(2):423–36.
5. Gerdsen M, Hundscheid TM, Boudewyns A, Van Rompaey V, Van De Berg R, Widdershoven JCC. Vestibular assessment in children with sensorineural hearing loss: diagnostic accuracy and proposal for a diagnostic algorithm. Front Neurol. 2024;1(15):1349554.
6. Wiener-Vacher SR, Wiener SI. Video head impulse tests with a remote camera system: normative values of semicircular canal vestibulo-ocular reflex gain in infants and children. Front Neurol. 2017;8:434.
7. Mittendorf N, et al. Test-retest reliability of the computerised rotational head impulse test in the pediatric population. Int J Otorhinolaryngol Head Neck Surg. 2023;9(1):5–11.
8. Basser L. Benign paroxysmal vertigo of childhood. Brain. 1964;87:141–52.
9. Carmona S, Sommerfleck PA, González Macchi ME, De Bagge MD, Áldez PC. Vestibular pathology in pediatric population; relevance of vestibular migraine. M J Pediatr. 2018;3:1–5.
10. Berg van de R, et al. Vestibular migraine and recurrent vertigo of childhood: diagnostic criteria consensus document of the Classification Committee of Vestibular Disorders of the Bárány Society and the International Headache Society. J Vestib Res. 2021;31(1):1–9.

4 Pharmacological Treatment of Vestibular Migraine in Children

Sudhira A. B. Ratnayake

4.1 Introduction

Migraine in children can be disabling and there are substantial differences with migraines in adults. Life-span population studies in USA indicate that in school-aged children, the average prevalence of migraines range from 8% to 24% [1]. Amongst this paediatric population, 0.6–1.8% of adolescents and 0.6% of children are estimated to have chronic migraine, where the child can have more than 15 days of headache per month, of which there are ≥8 days of migraine [2]. The same study reports that the rate of change in migraine for both sexes increased from age 3 years to the mid-20's [1]. Additionally, the authors indicate a bimodal distribution, peaking in the late teens to 20's and around 50 years of age. Such life-span epidemiological studies indicate the high prevalence of migraine in the paediatric population.

The Bárány Society has published its guidelines on diagnosis of paediatric vestibular migraine (VM) and recurrent vertigo of childhood [3]. This is based on clinical features and so far, there are no specific biomarkers that supports diagnosis. However, there can be associated co-morbidities and neurovestibular diagnostic abnormalities that includes pathological central oculomotor signs and subtle abnormal neuro-otological features [4, 5].

Compared to adults [2], it is well recognised that in children and adolescents, the symptom duration could be shorter than the 5 min to 72 h described by the Bárány Society criteria [3]. Hence, it is important to obtain a detailed anamnesis, preferably

S. A. B. Ratnayake (✉)
Department of Audio-Vestibular Medicine & Audiology, Alder Hey Children's NHS Foundation Trust, Liverpool, UK

School of Medicine, Faculty of Health and Life Sciences, University of Liverpool, Liverpool, UK

Postgraduate School of Medicine, NHS England, North West, UK
e-mail: sudhira.ratnayake@alderhey.nhs.uk

J. Saniasiaya (ed.), *Vestibular Migraine in Children and Adolescents: An overview*, https://doi.org/10.1007/978-981-96-2167-5_4

from the child's own descriptive vocabulary, which can be cross-checked with parents, to aid the diagnosis. This will enable the clinician to decide on a customised individual pharmacological and/or non-pharmacological treatment plan [6]. Some of these pharmacological agents may need to be prescribed and monitored under specialist follow-up.

Although some authors advocate non-pharmacological management is implemented first, the common consensus is that the combined pharmacological and non-pharmacological treatment would be far more effective at symptom control compared to pharmacological treatment alone [7].

4.2 Migraine and Vertigo Association

Basser's original publication in 1964 describes that benign paroxysmal vertigo of childhood is prevalent before the age 4 years and subsequently, symptom resolve by age 8–10 years [8]. The symptom descriptors include recurrent falls, inability to walk, self-perception of 'walls and ceiling falling over' and giddiness but there were no reported auditory symptoms. The onset could have been younger but often, such young pre-schoolers and toddlers may not be able to verbalise their symptoms. Therefore, their clinical presentations may go unreported. Often, the parents or carers may observe random, sudden onset and highly disturbed young child who may be crying and clutching at a parent or a surrounding object, in fear of the sudden rotatory vertiginous sensation. Therefore, clinicians would need to clarify the symptomatology and their temporal nature to ascertain the correct diagnosis.

Since early 1980s, this association between migraine, vertigo, and dizziness has been noted by several authors. Kayan and Hood [9] point out that significant more patients with migraine have vertigo compared to patients with tension-type headaches and Vuković and colleagues [10] describe similar associations compared with headache free controls.

The Headache Classification Committee of the International Headache Society (IHS), in their third edition, has recognised various 'childhood episodic syndromes' that may be associated with migraine [2]. Additional features include motion sickness, periodic sleep disturbances (including sleep walking and sleep talking), and bruxism. Hence, migraine and VM, with its vertigo and dizziness features, are now commonly accepted as closely associated with similar neuro-biological pathophysiology.

This close association between migraine and VM has led to the use of a range of pharmacological agents in VM that are generally effective in adults with migraines [11] and in children and adolescents with migraine [12].

Although headaches can be the dominant symptom in adults and in older adolescents with migraines, in paediatric VM, vestibular symptoms such as episodic dizziness, vertigo and imbalance or nausea and vomiting symptoms can be the dominant constellation of features [13]. Therefore, there may be a tendency for clinicians to treat children with antihistamines or anti-emetics [14]. On the other hand, as per the neuro-biological pathological mechanisms, clinicians may opt to treat the vertiginous migraines with standard headache-related migraine treatment options [5].

4.3 Factors to Consider in Paediatric Vestibular Migraine Treatment

4.3.1 Age, Gender and Pubertal Status

There is evidence of prevalence and clinical characteristic differences between males and females [15]. There appears to be a male/ female inversion of prevalence, where before puberty (before age 13 years), migraine prevalence is slightly higher in boys (29.4%) than in girls (25.6%). However, after puberty, it is commoner in females (12.7% in males versus 32.3% in females) [16]. Other authors have indicated that there is no significant difference between the migraine prevalence between girls and boys under 12 years of age [17].

An MRI study in children, with and without migraine aura, reports structural and functional brain differences in girls and boys compared with age- and sex-matched healthy controls [18]. These authors report that the sex differences in the brain regions are associated with sensory, motor and affective functions, providing an insight into the neural mechanisms related to differences in female migraine phenotype.

A control-matched longitudinal Swedish study, starting in 1955 and lasting 23 years, that recruited 73 children with migraine headaches and 73 control children without migraine, describes a prevalence of 1.4% at age7 years, gradually increasing to 5.3% at age 15 years [19]. The migraine group had a greater tendency to have abdominal pain, motion sickness, sleep disturbance and orthostatic symptoms. At puberty and as young adults, 62% were free from symptoms for at least 2 years. Of these, 22% had regular recurrence, indicating the fluctuating nature of the condition. The same study describes that 60% had classical migraine attacks at age 30 years and it was noted that girls had a greater relapse rate than boys. Therefore, features such as age, gender and pubertal status can be factors to consider when deciding on pharmacological treatment.

4.3.2 Family History, Inheritance and Genetic Factors

The above Swedish longitudinal study describes that every third family with a parent in the migraine group had at least one child over 4 years of age with migraine, indicating the strong first-degree family history for migraine [19]. Similarly, other studies conducted in twins and families in 1990s demonstrate a similar strong first-degree inherited in 35–60% [20, 21].

The complex genetic and environmental polygenic factors affecting the pathophysiology of migraine, and thus of vestibular migraine, is increasingly being recognised [22]. Currently, genomic-wide association studies have identified more than 180 monogenic variants belonging to complex networks of "pro-migraine" molecules in neuronal and vascular tissues [23].

The genomic studies and the functional imaging studies have identified the key mechanisms of the trigemino-vascular and vestibulo-thalamo-cortical dysfunction [24], along with the multimodal sensory and nociceptive dysmodulations [25] in the pathophysiology of vestibular migraine. Thus, these pathophysiological mechanisms and central neural regions would be the key targets for pharmacological therapeutics in vestibular migraine.

4.3.3 Frequency and Severity of Episodes

Generally, the frequency and severity of VM episodes will determine the start of pharmacological treatment. Viola and colleagues indicate that, in their experience, prophylaxis treatment should be started when there are more than three attacks per month or if symptoms are severe [14].

American Academy of Neurology (AAN) has published practice guidelines on acute and preventative treatments of paediatric migraines by considering numerous randomised controlled trials (RCTs) that evaluate both acute [26] and preventative [27] medication efficacies compared to placebo. AAN has considered the headache pain severity reduction for the efficacy in acute treatment whereas for preventative efficacy, AAN has considered a reduction of attack frequency.

4.3.4 Other Miscellaneous Factors

Langhagen and colleagues indicate that the selection of pharmacological agents should be based upon the co-morbidities [7]. If the child has asthma, medications such as beta-blockers are contraindicated. If there is obesity or if a child is overweight, then medications such as Pizotifen may need to be avoided.

Additionally, the treating clinician would need to listen to the preference of the child or the family, after discussion of the probable side effects of each medication.

Route of delivery and format of medication such as oral tablets, oral disintegrating tablets, oral solution (e.g., in younger children), nasal spray and transdermal patches are other reasons to consider when commencing pharmacological treatment.

Please see Table 4.1 for a summary of facors to consider when selecting pharmacological treatment in paediatric VM.

Table 4.1 Factors to consider in drug selection in paediatric vestibular migraine

Factors in drug selection
Age, gender and pubertal status
Frequency of attacks
Severity of attacks
Co-morbidities of the patient: e.g., 1. Asthma 2. Obesity
Side effects of the pharmacological agent
Patient or parent preference
Overlapping paediatric vertigo conditions: 1. Ménière's disease 2. Psychological features
Route and format of medication delivery, e.g. tablet, solution, injection, transdermal patch

4.4 Acute or Abortive Treatment

The main aim in acute or abortive treatment is to reduce the migraine headaches rapidly. However, abortive treatment should be for short durations and limited to two to three times a week [12], in order to avoid medication overuse headaches. Hence, these are generally advised to be used 'as and when required' (*PRN* or Pro re nata basis).

4.4.1 Pharmacological Pathophysiology of Acute Migraine

Functional imaging studies using positron emission tomography (PET) scans with triggered [28] and spontaneous [29] migraines have identified pontine, midbrain and hypothalamic activation. Hypothalamus has extensive central connections to the limbic system and these PET scan studies have identified activation of the hypothalamic area in the pre-monitory phase, giving rise to yawning, food craving and mood changes [28].

Denuelle and colleagues, in their PET scan study, have shown that a single Sumatriptan injection relieved the initial spontaneous migraine attack in less than 60 minutes post-dose [29].

In addition to the brainstem and hypothalamic region activation, the migraine headaches are associated with the trigeminal nerve activation and release of calcitonin gene-related peptide (CGRP) from the trigemino-vascular system [30].

4.4.1.1 Simple Analgesic Agents

If the acute VM presents with headache pains, most parents may resort to using over the counter (OTC) simple analgesia to achieve sufficient relief. These are well-tolerated with little or no side effects. A double-blind, randomized, placebo-controlled cross-over study has found that both Ibuprofen and Paracetamol (Acetaminophen) were more likely than a placebo to reduce the headache intensity 2 hours after treatment [31]. In fact, Ibuprofen is three times more likely than a placebo to abort migrainous headaches within 2 hours.

Other non-steroidal anti-inflammatory drugs (NSAIDs) can provide relief for migrainous pains. Naproxen is a prescription NSAID and it is approved by the United States Food and Drug Administration (FDA) to be used in combination with Sumatriptan in paediatric migraines. Naproxen is also available as an OTC format [12]. As they have an anti-inflammatory action, NSAIDs act on the nociceptors, pain pathways and central pain sensitisation mechanisms within the brain. Unlike narcotics, NSAIDS are not habit forming [32].

4.4.1.2 Triptans

Triptans have been studied extensively and it is thought to act by reversing blood vessel dilatation that occur in migraine. They are more effective if given in the early stages of the episode. Furthermore, spiral and vestibular ganglion cells express serotonin receptors (5-HT1A, 5-HT1B, 5-HT1D and 5-HT1F) and this is thought to explain the efficacy of triptans and ergots in VM [33, 34].

Sumatriptan was approved by FDA in 1992 and since then, triptans have been the leading pharmacological agent for acute migraine treatment [35].

As indicated earlier, as the triptans have a different action to that of NSAIDs, Sumatriptan is more effective when given in combination with an NSAID [32]. This combined action can be very effective in menstrual migraines as it acts on both the pain pathways (NSAID) and the suppression of vascular dilatation (triptan).

Triptans are generally given orally (enteral route) but Sumatriptan and Zolmitriptan are available as nasal sprays. This intranasal route is preferable for those patients that have significant nausea and vomiting.

The FDA has given approval for Almotriptan, Rizatriptan and combined Sumatriptan/ Naproxen for treatment of acute migraine in adolescents aged 12–17 years. Rizatriptan is additionally approved for use in children 6–11 years [12].

Children with episodic migraine appear to benefit from triptans than those with chronic migraines. Other features such as presence or absence of aura symptoms or autonomic symptoms does not appear to predict the triptan response [36].

There is mixed evidence for the use of many of the triptans:

- Sumatriptan is the most widely used triptan in adults. However, in paediatric population, a Japanese multi-centre double-blind RCT found no statistically significant difference in pain relief after 2 hours with oral sumatriptan compared to a placebo [37].
- On the other hand, Sumatriptan nasal spray given at a 20-mg dose provided greater rates of relief at 30 min and 2 hours after treatment compared to the placebo. It is well-tolerated in some adolescents [38].
- Compared to placebo treatment, there is high confidence of evidence that adolescents are likely to be free of acute headaches at 2 hours after taking oral Sumatriptan/ Naproxen and Zolmitriptan nasal spray [26].
- Zolmitriptan nasal spray provides fast pain relief after 15-minutes post-dose [39].
- Oral Zolmitriptan and Ibuprofen provide similar pain relief 2-hours post-dose compared to placebo [40].
- Rizatriptan, compared to placebo, appear to give relief from migraine headaches in children aged 6–17 years in a double-blind RCT [39].
- In adolescents, there appears to be a high placebo response rate, making it difficult to interpret the efficacy of available evidence [40].

Counselling for anticipated side effects from triptan prescription is important. These may include drowsiness, dizziness, tingling, chest tightness and serotonergic side effects [12]. Historically, triptans were contraindicated in those with increased vascular stroke risk. However, some smaller patient-cohort studies have found that triptans can be safely used in patients without a clear risk of vascular events [41, 42].

4.4.1.3 Ergotamine Derivatives

A non-triptan nasal spray Dihydroergotamine (ergotamine derivative) [43] is also available but there is evidence that it produces less effective relief of headache and nausea compared to Sumatriptan nasal spray [44].

Please see Table 4.2 for a summary of common pharmacological agents used in acute VM.

Table 4.2 Common drugs used in acute vestibular migraine

Pharmacological agent	Route/Age	Pharmacological action	Potential side effects
Ibuprofen	By mouth as immediate release/from 1 to 2 months By mouth as modified-release medications/from 12 to 17 years	Analgesia; anti-inflammatory	Constipation, gastrointestinal discomfort, haemorrhage, renal injury
Paracetamol (acetaminophen)	By mouth/from 1 to 2 months By rectum/from 1 to 2 months	Non-opioid analgesia; Anti-pyrexial	Agranulocytosis, hepatic function abnormalities, Bronchospasm
Naproxen/ Sumatriptan	By mouth	Anti-inflammatory and vasoconstriction (useful in menstrual migraines)	Cardiovascular and gastrointestinal effects
Sumatriptan	By mouth/from age 6 to 17 years By subcutaneous injection/from age 10 to 17 years By intranasal administration/ from age 12 to 17 years	Serotonin ($5HT_{1B/1D}$) agonist and vasoconstriction	Coronary vasospasms, ischaemic heart disease, hypertension, peripheral vascular disease
Zolmitriptan	By mouth/from age 12 to 17 years By intranasal administration/ from age 12 to 17 years	Serotonin receptor agonist	Arrhythmias, coronary vasospasms, peripheral vascular disease
Dihydroergotamine (ergotamine derivative)	FDA approved	Serotonin (or 5HT1D) agonist; intracranial vasoconstriction; inhibition of pro-inflammatory neuropeptide release from sensory nerves in the trigeminal system	Nausea

Note: Some information based on British National Formulary for Children (Reference: Paediatric Formulary Committee. *BNF for Children* (online). London: BMJ, Pharmaceutical Press, and RCPCH Publications. Available from: http://www.medicinescomplete.com. Accessed 23 June 2024)

4.4.2 Efficacy of Medications in Acute Migraine Treatment

According to the published guidelines of AAN, there are different levels of confidence on various pharmacological agents on controlling acute symptoms such as headache pains, nausea, vomiting, photophobia and phonophobia [26] (see Table 4.3).

- There is low or very low confidence in Sumatriptan nasal spray relieving headache pains at 30 min or at 1 hour, respectively [38].

Table 4.3 Acute migraine treatment: trial evidence confidence relative to placebo [26]

Outcome	High confidence (more likely than placebo)	Moderate confidence (probably more likely than placebo)	Low confidence (possibly more likely than placebo)
Headache pain-free at 1 hour	No evidence	Zolmitriptan Nasal Spray 5 mg	No evidence
Headache pain-free at 2 hours	Sumatriptan/ Naproxen oral tablet 10/60 mg Sumatriptan/ Naproxen oral tablet 30/180 mg Sumatriptan/ Naproxen oral tablet 85/500 mg Zolmitriptan Nasal Spray 5 mg	Ibuprofen Oral Solution 7.5—10 mg/kg Sumatriptan Nasal Spray 20 mg	Rizatriptan Oral Disintegrating Tablet 5—10 mg
Relief of nausea or vomiting at 2 hours	No evidence	No evidence	No evidence
Relief of photophobia at 30 min	No evidence	Zolmitriptan Nasal Spray 5 mg	No evidence
Relief of photophobia at 2 hours	No evidence	Sumatriptan/Naproxen Oral tablet 10/60 mg Sumatriptan/Naproxen Oral tablet 85/500 mg	Zolmitriptan Nasal Spray 5 mg
Relief of phonophobia at 30 min	No evidence	Zolmitriptan Nasal Spray 5 mg	No evidence
Relief of phonophobia at 2 hours	No evidence	Sumatriptan/Naproxen Oral tablet 10/60 mg Sumatriptan/Naproxen Oral tablet 85/500 mg	Sumatriptan Nasal Spray 5 mg Sumatriptan Nasal Spray 20 mg Sumatriptan/Naproxen Oral tablet 30/180 mg

- However, clinical trials using Sumatriptan/ Naproxen oral tablets [45, 46] and Zolmitriptan Nasal spray [47, 48] can relieve the headache pains by 2 hours in comparison to placebo treatment. Hence, patients may need to be counselled on the approximate time by which they are expected to get better.
- There were no medications with high, moderate or low confidence, compared to placebo, that relieved nausea or vomiting within 2 hours [26]. Hence, if this is a co-existing symptom, then the clinician may consider anti-emetic medications.
- The AAN guidelines also indicate moderate or low confidence in trial outcomes in alleviating photophobia and phonophobia at 30 min and 2 hours [45, 47].

Some RCTs prior to 2000 indicate that in about 1/3 of young migraineurs, symptomatic treatment of acute migraine with analgesics and NSAIDs may not be effective [49] but in the last 2 decades, emulating encouraging results in adults, triptan based medication trials, such as Sumatriptan nasal spray, has been found to be effective in paediatric acute migraine [50, 51].

4.5 Prophylactic Treatment

Various classes of medications have been used for preventative treatment of migraine and thus for VM. Common prophylactic agents used in paediatric migraine such as Propranolol, Topiramate, Pizotifen, Amitriptyline and Gabapentin [52] can be used in prophylactic treatment of childhood VM. Similar to the treatment of acute episodes, the aim in prophylaxis is to relieve the severity and frequency of the VM episodes. Some authors recommend considering start of prophylactic medication if there are more than one episode per week [12].

Counselling the patient and family, prior to starting medications, is essential. Families should be advised on the need for regular daily use of medication, rather than sporadic use, to help reduce the severity and frequency of the episodes. In chronic migraine situations, a reasonable goal would be to reduce the frequency and severity by 50% [12]. In addition to pharmacological treatment, other non-pharmacological strategies may need to be considered on a case-by-case basis to achieve greater successful outcomes.

The outcome evidence for paediatric migraine management is sparse and limited to small studies. Hence, they are largely extrapolated from research done in adults. Childhood and Adolescent Migraine Prevention (CHAMP) study was a multicentre, double-blinded placebo-controlled trial with a recruitment target of 675 subjects between ages 8 and 17 years with migraine, with or without aura, or chronic migraine, to study the effectiveness between Amitriptyline, Topiramate and a placebo with a primary outcome aim of reducing the headache frequency by 50% or more between 28 days from the start and last 28 days of a 24 week trial [53].

The CHAMP study eventually recruited 361 patients who were randomised to receive Amitriptyline (132), Topiramate (130) and the placebo (66). However, it was concluded early due to futility during interim analysis as there was no difference between the groups. The trial study reports adverse effects such as fatigue, dry mouth and altered mood in the Amitriptyline group and Paraesthesia and weight loss in the Topiramate group [54].

Other authors have queried the reasons for the high placebo response rate and highlight the unintentional non-pharmacological positive biopsychosocial feedback received by the CHAMP participants as they had very frequent clinical contact via 8 in-person visits over the 24-week period (approximately one contact every 3–4 weeks) during the drug delivery phase [55]. This is in keeping with the Cochrane systematic review of the positive benefit of frequent follow-ups in health conditions with chronic pain in children and adolescents, where more positive benefit is associated with in-person follow-ups [56] than from remote consultations [57]. Furthermore, it also highlights the importance of using both pharmacological and non-pharmacological therapeutic options in migraine disorders.

Treating clinicians may also consider pharmacological agents to control nausea and vomiting. Hence, in addition to the primary migraine prophylactic agent, a variety of adjunctive anti-emetics, especially in acute attacks or in in breakthrough episodes, can be used [58]. Some antihistamines may in fact, be targeting specific histamine receptors that are key to the pathophysiology of vestibular migraines [14].

The dose of prophylactic agents such as Topiramate, Amitriptyline and beta-blockers (Propranolol or Metoprolol) can be raised in incremental fashion, especially to titrate with the symptom frequency and severity in the 8-to-12-week follow-up period after the start of the medication [7].

Additionally, Langhagen and colleagues suggest that the pharmacological prophylaxis can be maintained until a sustained symptom titration occurs over a 4–6 months period. It can then be reduced or weaned off gradually over an 8-to-12-week period [7].

Additional pharmacological agents can be used to control nausea and vomiting. Hence, in addition to the primary migraine prophylactic agent, a variety of adjunctive anti-emetics, especially in acute attacks or in breakthrough episodes, can be used [58]. Some antihistamines may in fact, be targeting specific histamine receptors that are key to the pathophysiology of vestibular migraine [14].

4.5.1 Serotonin Modulators

Pizotifen is a serotonin and histamine antagonist and is one of the oldest anti-migraine drugs. RCTs involving Pizotifen, many in adults [59] and a few in paediatric age groups [60], were carried out in 1970s and 1980s. These indicate that Pizotifen is superior to a placebo and is not inferior to Naproxen, Flunarizine, Valproate or Clonidine.

Lawrence et al. (1977) [61], in their placebo-controlled trial in 37 children (6–15 years) at a dosage of 1.5 mg/day states a significant reduction in the frequency of the episodes with mild side effects such as nausea and vomiting, probably related to the primary migraine condition itself. A subsequent double-blind placebo-controlled cross-over RCT by Gillies et al. (1986), carried out in 7–14 years old children, indicates no difference between the active medication and placebo [62]. Common side effects, across research trials and in clinical practice, include weight gain, increased appetite and drowsiness [60, 62].

Although not available in the USA [63, 64], Pizotifen is widely used in Europe, including UK (Martin, 2020 abstract). It is relatively inexpensive and thus can be an affordable and an effective migraine preventive drug across many nations [59].

4.5.2 Anticonvulsants

Cortical spreading depression wave has been proposed as an integral pathophysiological mechanism in migraine [64] where there is a slowly propagating wave of cortical neural hyperexcitation followed by a period of neuronal inhibition, that results in tiredness [65, 66]. In its aftermath, there is activation of meningeal nociceptors, resulting in headaches, via the extracellular release of potassium ions, hydrogen ions and glutamate. This causes an axonal reflex leading to release of vasoactive neuropeptides such as substance P and calcitonin gene-related peptide (CGRP) [65]. Repeated or continued discharge cause sensitisation of trigeminovascular neural networks. The general role of anti-epileptic pharmaceutical drugs is to act on voltage and receptor-gated channels to reduce the release of these vasoactive neuropeptides and thus, stabilise neuronal membrane, leading to blocking the central spreading depression and prevent cortical neural sensitisation [66, 67].

Related to the side effects, in general, anti-epileptics medications are associated with teratogenicity [68] and hence, in appropriate adolescents of child-bearing age, the treating clinician needs to discuss this potential side effect.

4.5.2.1 Topiramate

Current literature indicates that Topiramate is the best studied prophylactic agent in children with migraines [12, 27]. In a single-centre, double-blind, placebo-controlled trial with a total of 44 children with migraine, the children were randomised in equal numbers to receive the active drug and the placebo [69]. Theses children were treated for a total duration of 4 months and in the first 4 weeks, Topiramate was titrated weekly in 25 mg increments to 100 mg/day in two divided doses or to the maximum tolerated dose. The study reports a statistically significant decrease in the Paediatric Migraine Disability Assessment Scale (PedMIDAS) and in school absenteeism in those taking Topiramate compared to the placebo. Side effects included weight loss, decreased concentration in school and paraesthesia but these were mild to moderate and did not cause drop out from the study.

A further double-blind, placebo-controlled Topiramate study in 12–17-year-olds over a 12-week period found that Topiramate 100 mg per day dose statistically significantly reduced the monthly migraine episode frequency [70]. The authors report more upper respiratory infections, paraesthesia and dizziness more commonly occurring in the active drug group.

Other side effects of Topiramate, such as reducing appetite and inducing weight loss [71], are thought to have beneficial effects in obese or overweight adolescents and is even suggested as a factor to discuss with the child to promote the use of Topiramate to reduce migraine severity [72]. It has been suggested that the clinician can thus cautiously approach this secondary goal of losing weight as a benefit in using Topiramate [73].

A recent meta-analysis identifies that Topiramate can significantly reduce the monthly migraine-related negative effects in children under 18 years [74]. The authors recognise that adverse effects are more frequent and hence, treating clinicians should discuss potential adverse effects with the child and the family, taking into consideration other co-morbidities such as overweight or obese body status of the patient.

If a patient tolerates Topiramate for 1–2 months, it is recommended that it is continued for at least 6 months prior to medication tapering or discontinuation [75, 76]. If there is recurrence after an attempted tapering, it should be re-introduced and continued for another 6 months before reconsidering a further tapering.

4.5.2.2 Sodium Valproate (Divalproex Sodium)

The active component in Sodium valproate is Valproic Acid (VPA) that readily crosses into the central nervous system within minutes of administration [64, 77]. Although the mechanism of VPA action is not fully understood, it is thought to increases the neuro-inhibitory action of Gamma Amino Butyric Acid (GABA) and thus potentiate its postsynaptic activities. VPA also inhibits N-methyl-D-aspartate or NMDA-evoked neuroexcitatory signals. NMDA receptors are glutamate receptors. These actions are believed to play a role in blocking the 'central spreading depression' wave [78]. At high doses, VPA increase extracellular Serotonin and Dopamine and their metabolites [79].

Studies have shown that VPA is at least as equally effective as Propranolol [80]. Sodium valproate generally gets rapidly absorbed, with peak concentrations occurring in 1–4 h [77]. A common side effect of VPA is weight gain [12].

4.5.2.3 Levetiracetam

This pharmacological agent targets hyperexcitable neurons that actively release neurotransmitters. By binding to the synaptic vesicle protein, this blocks further neurotransmitter release [64]. It is well-tolerated and the common side effects include irritability and hyperactivity.

4.5.2.4 Gabapentin

This acts by blocking the voltage-gated calcium channel receptors, thus reducing the transduction of membrane potential changes [81]. Additionally, it blocks vasoactive neuropeptide release and inhibit neuroexcitatory glutamate. The evidence for its efficacy is insufficient and is not indicated as a primary therapy. Its main side effects are fatigue, nausea and somnolence [82].

4.5.2.5 Carbamazepine

Carbamazepine binds and inhibit voltage-gated sodium channels and can contribute to increase extracellular serotonin [83].

4.5.3 Beta-Blockers

Beta-blockers such as Propranolol and Metoprolol can be used in the prophylaxis of migraine disorders in children. In a double-blind cross-over study over a 26-week period, in a cohort of 7–16 year olds (18 boys and 14 girls), Propranolol was noted to possibly more likely to achieve a 50% reduction in migraine headaches compared to those on placebo [84]. It is available as an oral solution and is licenced for use from age 2 years onwards [85] and hence, can be used in very young children when they present with benign paroxysmal vertigo which is considered as an early migraine variant [86].

Beta-blockers are contraindicated in patients with asthma. Propranolol can also cause bradycardia and hypotension in higher doses [12].

4.5.4 Calcium Channel Blockers

Flunarizine is not available in the United States but is available in Canada [27] and in European states. The practice guidelines of the AAN [27] indicate that there is insufficient evidence to determine whether Flunarizine, when compared to a placebo, would reduce the migraine attacks [87].

4.5.5 Antidepressants

The main side effect of antidepressants such as Amitriptyline is drowsiness but this can be minimised by giving the doses at bedtime in the night [12]. This has an additional advantage as those with migraine disorders who have a poor sleep pattern can trigger and worsen the migraine phenotype. Less commonly, cardiac rhythm abnormalities (prolonged QT interval) have been noted and hence, some clinicians carry out a screening ECG prior to starting Amitriptyline [12]. Hence, a cardiac history, including enquiring about palpitations, would be recommended.

4.5.6 Riboflavin

A double-blind, randomized, placebo-controlled study has concluded that high-dose Riboflavin can be a safe, well-tolerated and cost-effective prophylactic agent in migrainous children [88]. Half-life of riboflavin is about 1–2 hours and its absorption has is shown to reach saturation rate at 30–50 mg [89]. Therefore, in paediatric migraine patients, Riboflavin doses of 100–400 mg daily appear to be safe for several months [90].

4.5.7 Magnesium

Magnesium is involved in energy-consuming pathways and molecules in the body such as in protein synthesis, muscle contraction, cardiac excitability, glycolysis, hormonal synthesis and in the production of many human enzymes [91]. Magnesium-ATP complexes regulate cellular membrane channels such as sodium-potassium and calcium channels. Therefore, magnesium deficiency reduces cellular membrane resting potentials giving rise to hyper-excitability of neural pathways. Thus, magnesium plays a role in the cortical spreading depression in the central nervous system [92]. Thus, oral and intravenous magnesium has been used in migraine episodes.

A MEDLINE review in 2021 on Magnesium treatment in paediatric migraine has identified four studies in children from age 3 years to 17 years [93]. Although there was heterogeneity among the study designs in this review, the authors have identified that supplementary Magnesium in children can reduce the migraine headache frequency and severity. However, the optimal dosage, duration and route of administration remains unclear. Doses of up to 9 mg/kg/day of Magnesium oxide, along with adjunctive simple analgesia for 3–6 months, appear to be well-tolerated.

4.5.8 Betahistine

Betahistine, a histamine analogue, is a licenced medication in Meniere's disease-like symptom complexes [94]. Hence, when there are overlapping symptoms of Ménière and Migraine, especially in teenage age groups, the clinician may consider using this for long-term use.

4.5.9 CGRP Monoclonal Antibodies

Calcitonin gene-related peptide (CGRP) is a neurotransmitter produced in hypothalamus, cerebellum, brainstem and the trigeminal ganglion. It is a nociceptive transmitter and a strong vasodilator [12]. Goadsby and colleagues reports that plasma CGRP levels increase during migraine episodes but triptans reduce CGRP during migraine episodes [95, 96].

This is a novel type of treatment specifically developed for prevention of migraines [97] and is available as subcutaneous injections, mainly for adults.

Please see Table 4.4 for a summary of common prophylactic medications used in paediatric migrine.

Table 4.4 Common prophylactic drugs in paediatric migraine

Pharmacological agent	Route/age	Pharmacological action	Potential side effects
Pizotifen	By mouth/from age 5 years	Precise mechanism not known, probably inhibit serotonin and histamine receptors	Increased appetite, weight gain, drowsiness, sleepiness, tiredness
Topiramate	By mouth/from age 6 years	Anticonvulsant, mood stabiliser	Distal paraesthesia, loss of appetite, weight loss, anxiety
Sodium valproate	By mouth or rectum/from age 1 month	Precise mechanism not known, probably acting via GABA receptors	Hepatic dysfunction, Teratogenic, contraindicated in acute porphyria or suspected/ known mitochondrial disorders
Levetiracetam	By mouth/from age 1 month	Anticonvulsant	Anxiety, decreased appetite, behaviour abnormalities
Gabapentin	By mouth/from age 2 years	Anticonvulsant, Neuropathic pain, Anxiolytic	Sleepiness, Dizziness, suicidal ideation
Carbamazepine	By mouth using immediate release medicines/from age 1 month	Anticonvulsant, Neuropathic pain	Dizziness, drowsiness, dry mouth
Propranolol	By mouth/from age 2 years	Antihypertensive, Anxiolytic	Nausea, abdominal pain, constipation, contraindicated in asthma
Flunarizine	By mouth/from age 3 years as per small RCTs (2.5—10 mg/day)	Reduce arterial and arteriolar smooth muscle vasospasm	Hypotension, heart failure, arrythmia, low mood, contraindicated in depression
Amitriptyline	By mouth/from age 2 years	Neuropathic pain	Dry mouth, drowsiness, dizziness, glaucoma
Riboflavin (vitamin B_2)	By mouth/from neonatal period	Various mechanisms including reducing neuroinflammation and neuropathic pain	Urine discolouration
Magnesium	By mouth/from age 2–3 years	Alter nociceptor and neurotransmitter release	Nausea, vomiting, flushing
CGRP monoclonal antibodies	By subcutaneous injections/for adults	Block CGRP receptors and affect neurotransmission	Mild injection site reactions (pain, swelling and skin reaction), constipation

4.6 Limitations in Pharmacology Studies in Paediatric Migraine Disorders

Some clinical trials have conflicting results [27, 98]. These conflicting results in RCTs in children for the efficacy of preventative migraine medications are mainly due to improvement of frequency and severity of migraine attacks in the placebo arm of the RCT [99]. Evers and colleagues [100] also indicate that age and sex do not play a major role in the placebo response and are not important factors in RCT design. They further indicate that larger sample size and multi-centre designs, as opposed to single-centre studies, are factors associated with higher placebo responses.

Therefore, there are only few clinical RCTs conducted for acute and preventative [98] pharmacological treatment of VM in the paediatric population.

4.7 Conclusions

A variety of pharmacological agents can be used to treat both acute and preventative phases of paediatric VM. The evidence for such pharmacological therapeutics come from the adult and paediatric migraine studies. There is a strong association between migraine and VM and both share common pathophysiological mechanisms. A variety of pharmacological studies and clinical trials have shown varying degrees of statistically proven efficacy with conflicting evidence in some instances. Therefore, clinicians may consider both pharmacological and non-pharmacological treatment options to treat paediatric VM.

References

1. Victor T, Hu X, Campbell J, Buse D, Lipton R. Migraine prevalence by age and sex in the United States: a life-span study. Cephalalgia. 2010;30(9):1065–72. https://doi.org/10.1177/0333102409355601.
2. International Headache Society. Headache Classification Committee of the International Headache Society (IHS) the international classification of headache disorders, 3rd edition. Cephalalgia. 2018;38(1):1–211. https://doi.org/10.1177/0333102417738202.
3. Van de Berg R, Widdershoven J, Bisdorff A, et al. Vestibular migraine and recurrent vertigo of childhood: diagnostic criteria consensus document of the Classification Committee of Vestibular Disorders of the Bárány Society and the International Headache Society. J Vestib Res. 2021;31(1):1–9. https://doi.org/10.3233/VES-200003.
4. Crunkhorn R, Ratnayake S, Dasgupta S. Vestibular migraine in children [British Paediatric Neurology Association abstract 1747]. Arch Dis Child. 2021;106(Suppl 1) https://doi.org/10.1136/archdischild-2021-rcpch.826.
5. Viola P, Scarpa A, Chiarella G, et al. Instrumental assessment and pharmacological treatment of migraine-related vertigo in pediatric age. Audiol Res. 2024;14(1):129–38. https://doi.org/10.3390/audiolres14010011.
6. Iannone LF, De Cesaris F, Geppetti P. Emerging pharmacological treatments for migraine in the pediatric population. Life (Basel). 2022;12(4):536. https://doi.org/10.3390/life12040536.

7. Langhagen T, Landgraf MN, Huppert D, Heinen F, Jahn K. Vestibular migraine in children and adolescents. Curr Pain Headache Rep. 2016;20:67. https://doi.org/10.1007/s11916-016-0600-x.
8. Basser LS. Benign paroxysmal vertigo of childhood: a variety of vestibular neuronitis. Brain. 1964;87:141–52.
9. Kayan A, Hood JD. Neuro-otological manifestations of migraine. Brain. 1984;107(4):1123–42. https://doi.org/10.1093/brain/107.4.1123.
10. Vuković V, Plavec D, Galinović I, Lovrenčić-Huzjan A, Budišić M, Demarin V. Prevalence of vertigo, dizziness, and migrainous vertigo in patients with migraine. Headache. 2007;47(10):1427–35. https://doi.org/10.1111/j.1526-4610.2007.00939.x.
11. Bisdorff AR. Management of vestibular migraine. Ther Adv Neurol Disord. 2011;4:183–91. https://doi.org/10.1177/1756285611401647.
12. Merison K, Jacobs H. Diagnosis and treatment of childhood migraine. Curr Treat Options Neurol. 2016;18:11. https://doi.org/10.1007/s11940-016-0431-4.
13. Gruber M, Cohen-Kerem R, Kaminer M, Shupak A. Vertigo in children and adolescents: characteristics and outcome. Sci World J. 2012;2012:1–6. https://doi.org/10.1100/2012/109624.
14. Viola P, Marcianò G, Casarella A, et al. The pharmacological treatment of pediatric vertigo. Children (Besel). 2022;9(5):584. https://doi.org/10.3390/children9050584.
15. Ursitti F, Valeriani M. Migraine in childhood: gender differences. Eur J Paediatr Neurol. 2023;42:122–5. https://doi.org/10.1016/j.ejpn.2023.01.002.
16. Slater S, Crawford M, Kabbouche M, et al. Effects of gender and age on paediatric headache. Cephalalgia. 2009;29(9):969–73. https://doi.org/10.1111/j.1468-2982.2008.01827.x.
17. Genizi J, Khourieh Matar A, Zelnik N, Schertz M, Srugo I. Frequency of pediatric migraine with aura in a clinic-based sample. Headache. 2016;56(1):113–7. https://doi.org/10.1111/head.12741.
18. Faria V, Erpelding N, Lebel A, et al. The migraine brain in transition: girls vs boys. Pain. 2015;156(11):2212–21. https://doi.org/10.1097/j.pain.0000000000000292.
19. Bille B. Migraine in childhood and its prognosis. Cephalalgia. 1981;1(2):71–5. https://doi.org/10.1111/j.1468-2982.1981.tb00012.x.
20. Russell MB, Hilden J, Sorensen SA, Olesen J. Familial occurrence of migraine without aura and migraine with aura. Neurology. 1993;43(7):1369. https://doi.org/10.1212/wnl.43.7.1369.
21. Russell MB, Olesen J. Increased familial risk and evidence of genetic factor in migraine. BMJ. 1995;311(7004):541–4. https://doi.org/10.1136/bmj.311.7004.541.
22. Pietrobon D, Moskowitz MA. Pathophysiology of migraine. Annu Rev Physiol. 2013;75(1):365–91. https://doi.org/10.1146/annurev-physiol-030212-183717.
23. Grangeon L, Lange KS, Waliszewska-Prosół M, et al. Genetics of migraine: where are we now? J Headache Pain. 2023;24:1. https://doi.org/10.1186/s10194-023-01547-8.
24. Espinosa-Sanchez JM, Lopez-Escamez JA. New insights into pathophysiology of vestibular migraine. Front Neurol. 2015:6. https://doi.org/10.3389/fneur.2015.00012.
25. Goadsby PJ, Charbit AR, Andreou AP, Akerman S, Holland PR. Neurobiology of migraine. Neuroscience. 2009;161(2):327–41. https://doi.org/10.1016/j.neuroscience.2009.03.019.
26. Oskoui M, Pringsheim T, Holler-Managan Y, et al. Practice guideline update summary: acute treatment of migraine in children and adolescents. Neurology. 2019;93(11):487–99. https://doi.org/10.1212/wnl.0000000000008095.
27. Oskoui M, Pringsheim T, Billinghurst L, et al. Practice guideline update summary: pharmacologic treatment for pediatric migraine prevention. Neurology. 2019;93(11):500–9. https://doi.org/10.1212/wnl.0000000000008105.
28. Maniyar FH, Sprenger T, Monteith T, Schankin C, Goadsby PJ. Brain activations in the premonitory phase of nitroglycerin-triggered migraine attacks. Brain. 2014;137(Pt 1):232–41. https://doi.org/10.1093/brain/awt320.
29. Denuelle M, Fabre N, Payoux P, Chollet F, Geraud G. Hypothalamic activation in spontaneous migraine attacks. Headache. 2007:1418–26. https://doi.org/10.1111/j.15264610.2007.00776.x.

30. Edvinsson L, Villalón CM, MaassenVanDenBrink A. Basic mechanisms of migraine and its acute treatment. Pharmacol Ther. 2012;136(3):319–33. https://doi.org/10.1016/j.pharmthera.2012.08.011.
31. Hämäläinen ML, Hoppu K, Valkeila E, Santavuori P. Ibuprofen or acetaminophen for the acute treatment of migraine in children: a double-blind, randomized, placebo-controlled, crossover study. Neurology. 1997;48(1):103–7. https://doi.org/10.1212/wnl.48.1.103.
32. Tepper DE. Non-steroidal anti-Inflammatories for the acute treatment of migraine. Headache. 2012;53(1):225–6. https://doi.org/10.1111/j.1526-4610.2012.02293.x.
33. Ahn SK, Balaban CD. Distribution of 5-HT1B and 5-HT1D receptors in the inner ear. Brain Res. 2010;1346:92–101. https://doi.org/10.1016/j.brainres.2010.05.057.
34. Balaban CD, Jacob RG, Furman JM. Neurologic bases for comorbidity of balance disorders, anxiety disorders and migraine: neurotherapeutic implications. Expert Rev Neurother. 2011;11(3):379–94. https://doi.org/10.1586/ern.11.19.
35. Zobdeh F, Kraiem A, Attwood MM, et al. Pharmacological treatment of migraine: drug classes, mechanisms of action, clinical trials and new treatments. Br J Pharmacol. 2021;178(23):4588–607. https://doi.org/10.1111/bph.15657.
36. Johnson HF, Goadsby PJ, Gelfand AA. Predictors of Triptan response in pediatric migraine. Pediatr Neurol. 2016;58:37–40. https://doi.org/10.1016/j.pediatrneurol.2016.01.022.
37. Fujita M, Sato K, Nishioka H, Sakai F. Oral sumatriptan for migraine in children and adolescents: a randomized, multicenter, placebo-controlled, parallel group study. Cephalalgia. 2014;34(5):365–75. https://doi.org/10.1177/0333102413510213.
38. Winner P, Rothner AD, Wooten JD, Webster C, Ames M. Sumatriptan nasal spray in adolescent migraineurs: a randomized, double-blind, placebo-controlled, acute study. Headache. 2006;46(2):212–22. https://doi.org/10.1111/j.1526-4610.2006.00339.x.
39. Ho TW, Pearlman E, Lewis D, et al. Efficacy and tolerability of rizatriptan in pediatric migraineurs: results from a randomized, double-blind, placebo-controlled trial using a novel adaptive enrichment design. Cephalalgia. 2012;32(10):750–65. https://doi.org/10.1177/0333102412451358.
40. Sun H, Bastings E, Temeck J, et al. Migraine therapeutics in adolescents: a systematic analysis and historic perspectives of triptan trials in adolescents. JAMA Pediatr. 2013;167(3):243. https://doi.org/10.1001/jamapediatrics.2013.872.
41. Klapper J, Mathew N, Nett R. Triptans in the treatment of basilar migraine and migraine with prolonged Aura. Headache. 2001;41(10):981–4. https://doi.org/10.1046/j.1526-4610.2001.01192.x.
42. Mathew P, Krel R, Buddhdev B, et al. A retrospective analysis of Triptan and DHE use for basilar and hemiplegic migraine. Headache. 2016;56(5):841–8. https://doi.org/10.1111/head.12804.
43. Silvestro M, Orologio I, Tessitore A, Trojsi F, Tedeschi G, Russo A. Dihydroergotamine mesylate nasal spray: an acute treatment option for migraine in adults. Expert Rev Neurother. 2024;24(6):1–10. https://doi.org/10.1080/14737175.2024.2342446.
44. Boureau F, Kappos L, Schoenen J, Esperança P, Ashford E. A clinical comparison of Sumatriptan nasal spray and Dihydroergotamine nasal spray in the acute treatment of migraine. Int J Clin Pract. 2000;54(5):281–6. https://doi.org/10.1111/j.17421241.2000.tb11905.x.
45. Derosier FJ, Lewis DW, Hershey AD, et al. Randomized trial of Sumatriptan and naproxen sodium combination in adolescent migraine. Pediatrics. 2012;129(6):e1411–20. https://doi.org/10.1542/peds.2011-2455.
46. Winner P, Linder S, Hershey AD. Consistency of response to Sumatriptan/naproxen sodium in a randomized placebo-controlled, cross-over study for the acute treatment of migraine in adolescence. Headache. 2015;55(4):519–28. https://doi.org/10.1111/head.12555.
47. Lewis DW, Winner P, Hershey AD, Wasiewski WW. Efficacy of Zolmitriptan nasal spray in adolescent migraine. Pediatrics. 2007;120(2):390–6. https://doi.org/10.1542/peds.2007-0085.
48. Winner P, Farkas V, Štillová H, et al. Efficacy and tolerability of zolmitriptan nasal spray for the treatment of acute migraine in adolescents: results of a randomized, double-blind,

multi-center, parallel-group study (TEENZ). Headache. 2016;56(7):1107–19. https://doi.org/10.1111/head.12859.
49. Hämäläinen ML, Hoppu K, Santavuori P. Sumatriptan for migraine attacks in children: a randomized placebo-controlled study. Do children with migraine respond to oral sumatriptan differently from adults? Neurology. 1997;48(4):1100–3. https://doi.org/10.1212/wnl.48.4.1100.
50. Callenbach PM, Pels LPM, Mulder PGH, et al. Sumatriptan nasal spray in the acute treatment of migraine in adolescents and children. Eur J Paediatr Neurol. 2007;11:325–30. https://doi.org/10.1016/j.ejpn.2007.02.010.
51. Major PW, Grubisa HIS, Thie NMR. Triptans for treatment of acute pediatric migraine: a systematic literature review. Pediatr Neurol. 2003;29(5):425–9. https://doi.org/10.1016/s0887-8994(03)00400-4.
52. Martin J. The preventative management of migraine headaches in paediatrics [neonatal and Paediatric pharmacists conference November 2019 abstract P29]. Arch Dis Child. 2020;105:e21. https://doi.org/10.1136/archdischild-2020-NPPG.38.
53. Hershey AD, Powers SW, Coffey CS, Eklund DD, Chamberlin LA, Korbee LL. Childhood and adolescent migraine prevention (CHAMP) study: a double-blinded, placebo-controlled, comparative effectiveness study of amitriptyline, topiramate, and placebo in the prevention of childhood and adolescent migraine. Headache. 2013;53(5):799–816. https://doi.org/10.1111/head.12105.
54. Powers SW, Coffey CS, Chamberlin LA, et al. Trial of amitriptyline, topiramate, and placebo for pediatric migraine. N Engl J Med. 2017;376(2):115–24. https://doi.org/10.1056/nejmoa1610384.
55. Nwaobi SE, Kamins J. Implications of 3-year follow-up data from the childhood and adolescent migraine prevention medication trial. JAMA Netw Open. 2021;4(7):e2114788. https://doi.org/10.1001/jamanetworkopen.2021.14788.
56. Fisher E, Law E, Dudeney J, Palermo TM, Stewart G, Eccleston C. Psychological therapies for the management of chronic and recurrent pain in children and adolescents. Cochrane Database Syst Rev. 2018;9:9. https://doi.org/10.1002/14651858.cd003968.pub5.
57. Fisher E, Law E, Dudeney J, Eccleston C, Palermo TM. Psychological therapies (remotely delivered) for the management of chronic and recurrent pain in children and adolescents. Cochrane Database Syst Rev. 2019;4:4. https://doi.org/10.1002/14651858.cd011118.pub3.
58. Shen Y, Qi X, Wan T. The treatment of vestibular migraine: a narrative review. Ann Indian Acad Neurol. 2020;23(5):602–7. https://doi.org/10.4103/aian.aian_591_19.
59. Fragoso YD, Lopes GCM, Santos GM, Carturan P, Martimbianco ALC. Pizotifen for the treatment of migraine: a systematic review and meta-analysis. Headache Med. 2021;12(3):168–81. https://doi.org/10.48208/HeadacheMed.2021.31.
60. Papetti L, Ursitti F, Moavero R, et al. Prophylactic treatment of pediatric migraine: is there anything new in the last decade? Front Neurol. 2019;10:771. https://doi.org/10.3389/fneur.2019.00771.
61. Lawrence ER, Hossain M, Littlestone W. Sanomigran for migraine prophylaxis; controlled multicenter trial in general practice. Headache. 1997;17:109–11. https://doi.org/10.1111/j.1526-4610.1977.hed1703109.x.
62. Gillies D, Sills M, Forsythe I. Pizotifen (Sanomigran) in childhood migraine: a double-blind controlled trial. Eur Neurol. 1986;25:32–5. https://doi.org/10.1159/000115983.
63. Lauritsen CG, Marmura MJ. Current treatment options: vestibular migraine. Curr Treat Options Neurol. 2017;19(11):38. https://doi.org/10.1007/s11940-017-0476-z.
64. Parikh SK, Silberstein SD. Current status of antiepileptic drugs as preventive migraine therapy. Curr Treat Options Neurol. 2019;21:4. https://doi.org/10.1007/s11940-019-0558-1.
65. Bernstein C, Burstein R. Sensitization of the trigeminovascular pathway: perspective and implications to migraine pathophysiology. J Clin Neurol. 2012;8(2):89. https://doi.org/10.3988/jcn.2012.8.2.89.
66. White HS. Molecular pharmacology of topiramate: managing seizures and preventing migraine. Headache. 2005;45(s1):S48–56. https://doi.org/10.1111/j.1526-4610.2005.4501006.x.

67. Costa C, Tozzi A, Rainero I, et al. Cortical spreading depression as a target for anti-migraine agents. J Headache Pain. 2013;14:1. https://doi.org/10.1186/1129-2377-14-62.
68. Meadow R. Anticonvulsants in pregnancy. Arch Dis Child. 1991;66(1 Spec):62–5. https://doi.org/10.1136/adc.66.1_spec_no.62.
69. Lakshmi CVS, Singhi P, Malhi P, Ray M. Topiramate in the prophylaxis of pediatric migraine: a double-blind placebo-controlled trial. J Child Neurol. 2007;22(7):829–35. https://doi.org/10.1177/0883073807304201.
70. Lewis D, Winner P, Saper J, et al. Randomized, double-blind, placebo-controlled study to evaluate the efficacy and safety of topiramate for migraine prevention in pediatric subjects 12 to 17 years of age. Pediatrics. 2009;123(3):924–34. https://doi.org/10.1542/peds.2008-0642.
71. Young WB. Preventive treatment of migraine: effect on weight. Curr Pain Headache Rep. 2008;12(3):201–6. https://doi.org/10.1007/s11916-008-0035-0.
72. Hershey AD, Powers SW, Nelson TD, et al. Obesity in the pediatric headache population: a multicenter study. Headache. 2009;49(2):170–7. https://doi.org/10.1111/j.1526-4610.2008.01232.x.
73. Kumar R. Safety considerations in prescribing topiramate in adolescents. 2009. Comment in: Lakshmi CVS, Singhi P, Malhi P, Ray M. (authors) Topiramate in the prophylaxis of pediatric migraine: a double-blind placebo-controlled trial. https://publications.aap.org/pediatrics/article-abstract/123/3/924/71669/Randomized-Double-Blind-Placebo-Controlled-Study?redirectedFrom=fulltext. Accessed 23 June 2024.
74. Wu X, Zhang Y, Lu M, et al. The efficacy and safety of topiramate in the prevention of pediatric migraine: an update meta-analysis. Front Pediatr. 2020:8. https://doi.org/10.3389/fped.2020.00028.
75. Pascual J, el Berdei Y, Gómez-Sánchez JC. How many migraine patients need prolonged (>1 year) preventive treatment? Experience with topiramate. J Headache Pain. 2007;8(2):90–3. https://doi.org/10.1007/s10194-007-0351-x.
76. Diener HC, Agosti R, Allais G, et al. Cessation versus continuation of 6-month migraine preventive therapy with topiramate (PROMPT): a randomised, double-blind, placebo-controlled trial. Lancet Neurol. 2007;6(12):1054–62. https://doi.org/10.1016/s1474-4422(07)70272-7.
77. Silberstein SD. Divalproex sodium in headache: literature review and clinical guidelines. Headache. 1996;36(9):547–55. https://doi.org/10.1046/j.1526-4610.1996.3609547.x.
78. Holland P, Akerman S, Goadsby P. Cortical spreading depression-associated cerebral blood flow changes induced by mechanical stimulation are modulated by AMPA and GABA receptors. Cephalgia. 2010;30(5):519–27. https://doi.org/10.1111/j.1468-2982.2009.02021.x.
79. Cutrer F, Limmroth V, Moskowitz M. Possible mechanisms of valproate in migraine prophylaxis. Cephalalgia. 1997;17(2):93–100. https://doi.org/10.1046/j.1468-2982.1997.1702093.x.
80. Afshari D, Rafizadeh S, Rezaei M. A comparative study of the effects of low-dose topiramate versus sodium valproate in migraine prophylaxis. Int J Neurosci. 2012;122(2):60–8. https://doi.org/10.3109/00207454.2011.626908.
81. Perloff MD, Berlin RK, Gillette M, Petersile MJ, Kurowski D. Gabapentin in headache disorders: what is the evidence? Pain Med. 2015;17:162–71. https://doi.org/10.1111/pme.12931.
82. Silberstein S, Goode-Sellers S, Twomey C, Saiers J, Ascher J. Randomized, double-blind, placebo-controlled, phase II trial of gabapentin enacarbil for migraine prophylaxis. Cephalalgia. 2013;33(2):101–11. https://doi.org/10.1177/0333102412466968.
83. Dailey JW, Reith MEA, Steidley KR, Milbrandt JC, Jobe PC. Carbamazepine-induced release of serotonin from rat hippocampus in vitro. Epilepsia. 1998;39(10):1054–63. https://doi.org/10.1111/j.1528-1157.1998.tb01290.x.
84. Ludvigsson J. Propranolol used in prophylaxis of migraine in children. Acta Neurol Scand. 1974;50(1):109–15. https://doi.org/10.1111/j.1600-0404.1974.tb01350.x.
85. Joint Formulary Committee. Propranolol hydrochloride. British National Formulary (online). London: BMJ and Pharmaceutical Press. https://bnfc.nice.org.uk/drugs/propranolol-hydrochloride/. Accessed 23 June 2024

86. Gelfand AA. Episodic syndromes of childhood associated with migraine. Curr Opin Neurol. 2018;31(3):281–5. https://doi.org/10.1097/wco.0000000000000558.
87. Sorge F, Simone RD, Marano E, Nolano M, Orefice G, Carrieri P. Flunarizine in prophylaxis of childhood migraine: a double-blind, placebo-controlled, crossover study. Cephalalgia. 1988;8(1):1–6. https://doi.org/10.1046/j.1468-2982.1988.0801001.x.
88. Talebian A, Soltani B, Banafshe HR, Moosavi GA, Talebian M, Soltani S. Prophylactic effect of riboflavin on pediatric migraine: a randomized, double-blind, placebo-controlled trial. Electron Physician. 2018;10(2):6279–85. https://doi.org/10.19082/6279.
89. Zempleni J, Galloway JR, McCormick DB. Pharmacokinetics of orally and intravenously administered riboflavin in healthy humans. Am J Clin Nutr. 1996;63(1):54–66. https://doi.org/10.1093/ajcn/63.1.54.
90. Sparaco M, Feleppa M, Lipton R, Rapoport A, Bigal M. Mitochondrial dysfunction and migraine. Cephalalgia. 2006;26(4):361–72. https://doi.org/10.1111/j.1468-2982.2005.01059.x.
91. Messina A, Ciodaro F, Corvaia A, Liberto S, Marino C. Use of magnesium citrate in the prophylaxis of vestibular migraine in childhood.; 2022. https://audiologiaefoniatria.padovauniversitypress.it/system/files/papers/IJAP-2022-1-7.pdf. Accessed 23 June 2024.
92. Sun-Edelstein C, Mauskop A. Role of magnesium in the pathogenesis and treatment of migraine. Expert Rev Neurother. 2009;9(3):369–79. https://doi.org/10.1586/14737175.9.3.369.
93. Avery J, Etheridge L. Is high-dose magnesium supplementation helpful in adolescents with migraine? Arch Dis Child. 2021;106(10):1027–30. https://doi.org/10.1136/archdischild-2021-321980.
94. Adrion C, Fischer CS, Wagner J, Gürkov R, Mansmann U, Strupp M. Efficacy and safety of beahistine treatment in patients with Meniere's disease: primary results of a long term, multicentre, double blind, randomised, placebo controlled, dose defining trial (BEMED trial). BMJ. 2016;352:h6816. https://doi.org/10.1136/bmj.h6816.
95. Goadsby PJ, Edvinsson L, Ekman R. Vasoactive peptide release in the extracerebral circulation of humans during migraine headache. Ann Neurol. 1990;28(2):183–7. https://doi.org/10.1002/ana.410280213.
96. Goadsby PJ, Edvinsson L. The trigeminovascular system and migraine: studies characterizing cerebrovascular and neuropeptide changes seen in humans and cats. Ann Neurol. 1993;33(1):48–56. https://doi.org/10.1002/ana.410330109.
97. The Migraine Trust. Calcitonin Gene-Related Peptide (CGRP) monoclonal antibodies. The Migraine Trust (online). https://migrainetrust.org/live-with-migraine/healthcare/treatments/calcitonin-gene-related-peptide-monoclonal-antibodies/#:~:text=CGRP%20monoclonal%20antibodies. Accessed 24 June 2024.
98. El-Chammas KA, Keyes J, Thompson N, Vijayakumar J, Becher D, Jackson J. Comparative effectiveness meta-analysis of drugs for the prophylaxis of pediatric migraine headache. JAMA Pediatr. 2013;167(3):250–8. https://doi.org/10.1001/jamapediatrics.2013.508.
99. Faria V, Linnman C, Lebel A, Borsook D. Harnessing the placebo effect in pediatric migraine clinic. J Pediatr. 2014;165(4):659–65. https://doi.org/10.1016/j.jpeds.2014.06.040.
100. Evers S, Marziniak M, Frese A, Gralow I. Placebo efficacy in childhood and adolescence migraine: an analysis of double-blind and placebo-controlled studies. Cephalalgia. 2009;29(4):436–44. https://doi.org/10.1111/j.1468-2982.2008.01752.x.

Non-pharmacological Treatment of Vestibular Migraine in Children

5

Jeyasakthy Saniasiaya

5.1 Introduction

Pharmacological treatments may not always be effective and can have safety issues in children and adolescents. Non-pharmacological interventions (NPIs) have shown promising avenues in managing chronic health conditions, including VM in adults. NPIs are science-based and non-invasive interventions that aim to treat, prevent, or cure health problems [1]. NPIs encompass products, methods, programmes, or services related to biological or psychosocial processes [1].

Evidence on NPIs in managing VM in children and adolescents is still lacking, as this entity is relatively new, and research and studies around this topic are still emerging. This chapter will be based on published research on NPIs in migraine in paediatric and VM in adult populations.

Non-pharmacological treatment has been found to be more effective than pharmacological therapy [2]. Interestingly, more research and evidence are touting non-pharmacological treatment for various conditions in children, notably migraine [3, 4]. Youths participating in the Childhood and Adolescents Migraine Prevention (CHAMP) medication study reported a reduction in headache days and migraine-related disability 3-years post-trial, regardless of whether they received the pharmacotherapy or placebo [4].

Although studies and research representing the paediatric population with vestibular migraine are still lacking, non-pharmacological treatment in children and adults follows the same fundamental basis. Several NPIs that have shown promising results in addressing VM include:

J. Saniasiaya (✉)
Department of Otorhinolaryngology, Faculty of Medicine, Universiti Malaya, Kuala Lumpur, Wilayah Persekutuan Kuala Lumpur, Malaysia
e-mail: jeyasakthy@um.edu.my

J. Saniasiaya (ed.), *Vestibular Migraine in Children and Adolescents: An overview*, https://doi.org/10.1007/978-981-96-2167-5_5

1. Lifestyle modifications.
2. Vestibular rehabilitation.
3. Cognitive behavioural therapy.
4. Mindfulness therapy.
5. Non-invasive brain stimulation.

5.1.1 Lifestyle Modifications

Lifestyle modification has made great strides in improving VM in children and adolescents, as a healthy lifestyle is found to be the key to health. The available research on lifestyle modifications stresses a perfect balance between regular sleep, timely meals, sufficient hydration, reduced caffeine, tobacco, and alcohol consumption, moderate physical activity, and eliminating stress as much as possible [5]. With the advent of technology, reducing electronic screen exposure needs to be emphasised.

According to the Childhood and Adolescent Migraine Prevention (CHAMP) study, a healthy lifestyle has been found to limit the use of medications to only acute attacks. As a preventative measure, children and adolescents were prescribed adequate hydration, regular exercise, adequate sleep, and avoiding skipping meals [6].

Evidence is touting poor lifestyle habits that trigger or prolong headache or migraine attacks or frequency [7].

5.1.1.1 Dietary Modifications

Diet or food has been documented to have an effect on our sympathetic nervous system, glucose metabolism in the brain, nitric oxide release, modulation of neuropeptides, neuroreceptors and ion channels, vasodilation and inflammatory process [8].

Between 7% and 44% of adults and children with migraine have reported that a migraine attack was triggered by certain foods or drinks [9, 10]. An earlier survey that dates back to 1979 involving 120 children with migraine conducted in the United Kingdom reports that fasting (41%) and specific food (38%) triggered migraine attacks whereby cheese was the predominant culprit in 17% of the children, followed by cheese (16%) and citrus (5%) [11]. Nonetheless, a more recent study involving 102 children and adolescents shows chocolate was the most common dietary trigger [12].

Biochemical properties in particular foods are believed to cause migraine attacks. For example, chocolate contains phenylalanine, and cheese contains tyramine, which has vasoconstrictive properties that result in changes in cerebral blood flow and the production of norepinephrine from sympathetic nerve cells [13].

Traditionally, dietary modifications revolve around dietary adjustment through eliminating food items that have been believed to trigger VM episodes. Over the past few decades, caffeine, chocolates, processed meats, alcoholic beverages, including red wine, cheese, artificial sweeteners, caffeine, and MSG, have been linked to migraine triggers [14–16].

High-folate diet, low-fat diet, high omega-3 and low omega-6 fatty acid diets, ketogenic diet, Atkins diet, and low sodium diet are among dietary interventions that have shown promising results among the adult population with migraine [8, 17].

Studies reporting solely involving children and adolescents with vestibular migraine on the effect of diet and nutrition are not present. Most of the data present concerning diet and nutrition is on children with migraine, although we acknowledge that vestibular migraine and migraine may not be comparable.

5.1.2 Vestibular Rehabilitation

5.1.2.1 Introduction

VR is a promising avenue believed to be more sustainable than pharmacological treatment. Great strides have been made over the last years in conducting various research and creating VR protocols to suit different age groups, genders, and conditions. The fundamental basis of VR is the central mechanisms of neuroplasticity that concurrently accelerate vestibular compensation [18]. VR encompasses three main domains: adaptation, habituation, and substitution, which result in vestibular compensation.

VR has been shown to significantly improve the quality of life of patients with vestibular and balance disorders [19]. Cochrane Database Systematic review reported moderate to strong evidence of VR for improving function and reducing symptoms among patients with vestibular hypofunction [20]. VR has been found to desensitise the vestibular system and increase the vestibular-ocular reflex and vestibular-spinal reflex gains while paving a new alternative sense for postural instability [21].

The effectiveness of VR in various vestibular disorders, both in adults and children, has been well-established [22–26]. Similarly, the role of VR in patients with VM has gained attention as some studies advocate that VR can be more effective than pharmacological treatment [2]. Over the past decade, VR has shown promising results in patients with VM [25, 27–31], although most studies revolve around the adult population. VR, which is carried out concurrently with preventative medication, has shown significant improvements in adult patients with VM [25, 27, 29].

The role of VM in children and adolescents with VM remains scarce, possibly because VM in children has only recently gained attention. Nonetheless, good outcomes were reported among the small number of studies that are available on VR in children with migraine [32].

VR typically encompasses four different components of exercise that aim to reduce functional disability and overall impairment in patients with vestibular dysfunction: (1) Gaze stability exercise to improve gaze stability, (2) Habituation exercise-aimed at adjusting symptoms, (3) Exercise to improve gait and balance, and (4) Endurance exercise [33].

Adaptation exercises entail the alteration of neuronal response in relation to head movements. Besides alleviating symptoms, the main aim of adaptation exercise is to improve gaze and postural stability [34]. Adaptation exercise requires children to maintain focus on a target while moving the head in various directions. Habituation requires children to undergo repeated exposure to a provocative stimulus with the intention of reducing the symptoms. VR exercises are tailored according to each child's specific based on the specific triggering movements. Substitution includes the usage of other sensory cues (alternative strategy) to attain gaze stabilisation and postural stability. For example, both visual and somatosensory are used for gaze stabilisation and balance, central pre-programming and anticipatory response [34]. It is important to understand that when incorporating VR exercises in children, it is crucial to incorporate and consider the functional aspects such as motor development and balancing rather than solely focusing on improving individual vestibular deficit.

Each VR exercise needs to be individualised and must consider each child's critical developmental periods, individual ability, cooperation, and attention.

The success of VR is dependent on several factors which are believed to affect the recovery: (1) Timing of delivery of VR, (2) age of the patient and critical periods of development, (3) Environmental enrichment, (4) Reliance on vestibular on the multisensory integrative process, (5) patients individual motivation and commitment, (6) motor learning [35].

VR demonstrated significant improvement among VM patients who developed deconditioning, imbalance or visual dependence [36, 37]. 56% of VM patients with motion-induced symptoms reported improvement following VR [38].

5.1.2.2 Evidence of Outcome of VR on VM

Gottshall et al. 2005 published a study investigating the effect of VR in patients with VM, including adolescent patients. In his study, patients with VM were divided into four groups: (1) idiopathic migraine-associated dizziness; (2) idiopathic migraine-associated dizziness with benign positional vertigo; (3) posttraumatic migraine-associated dizziness; and (4) posttraumatic migraine-associated dizziness with benign positional vertigo. Participants in this study were aged between 11 and 56 years. All patients were also given preventative medication (Neurontin 100 mg twice daily). The author found significant improvement in all four groups. The mean time to achieve remission was 9.5 weeks (range of 4.9–16.3 weeks) [29].

Koc et al., in their study, demonstrated that patients with VM who received VR over 1.5 months showed significant improvement in both subjective and objective scores. Each patient received 18 sessions for 1.5 months, and the pre-and post-treatment Dizziness Handicap Inventory (DHI) score, Vestibular Disorders Activities of Daily Living Scale (VADL) score, frequency of dizziness and headache, and computerised dynamic posturography (CDP) were evaluated. It was interesting in this study that the postural stability was measured post-treatment which showed improvement [31].

5.1.2.3 Concurrent Use of VRT and Other Treatment

Whitney et al. reported significant improvement among patients with VM on prophylaxis medication compared to none [25, 27] following VR. Patients with VM have been shown to present with space and motion discomfort [22, 39], and the use of prophylaxis mediation aids these patients in tolerating increased VR activity [27].

Vitkovic et al. advocated on longer intervention and a more intensive therapy for patients with VM in order to achieve daily levels of symptom [40]. In their study, 36 participants (VM = 20, vestibular impairment (VI) = 16) were subjected to a 9-week customised VR programme, of which each patient had five therapy appointments occurring at initial 2, 5, 9 and 6 months. The subjective and physical performance outcomes measured at baseline, 9 weeks and 6 months showed that both VM and VI groups benefitted equally from rehabilitation [40].

5.1.2.4 Role of VRT in Migraine Variants

VR has been shown to improve the headache or migraine component of VM [30]. A study from Japan by Sugaya et al. included 251 participants, among which 28 patients had VM, 79 patients with tension-type headaches, and 144 patients without headaches. The participants were educated on VR exercises for 5 days and the outcome of VR was performed using the Dizziness Handicap Inventory (DHI), Headache Impact Test (HIT-6), Hospital Anxiety and Depression Scale (HADS), and Somatosensory Catastrophizing Scale (SSCS) as well as centre of gravity fluctuation measurement as an objective dizziness severity index. The authors found that the participants with VM and tension-type headache demonstrated significant improvement in the HIT-6 score with improvement of the DHI, HADS, SSCS, and the centre of gravity measurement following VR [30].

Wrisley et al. compared 30 patients with migraine with vestibular/balance disorders and patients with vestibular disorders who underwent a customised VR programme for 4.1 sessions (mean) over 3.3 months (mean). The authors reported significant improvements in both groups when evaluated using the Dizziness Handicap Inventory, the Activities-Specific Balance Confidence Scale, the Dynamic Gait Index, and the Timed Up AND Go Test, as well as the severity of their dizziness on an analogue scale of 0–100. Interestingly, participants with a history of migraine perceived they were more disabled and less confident in their ability to maintain balance in performing everyday activities compared to the participants with vestibular disorders [23].

5.1.2.5 Evidence of Role of VRT in Children

VR has shown significant improvement in children with vestibular disorders [34]. Children with VM demonstrating significant space and motion discomfort may benefit from combination treatment, especially with prophylaxis medication, to tolerate the exercises until the medication can be stopped.

So far, only one study has published the outcome of VR in children and adolescents with VM [32]. In a study by Shaabani et al. [32] children aged between 9 and 15 diagnosed with VM by paediatric neurologists were evaluated using dizziness handicap inventory (DHI), headache impact test-6, and headache frequency before and after VR. The children and adolescents included received home-based VR and were assessed after 1 month and found significant improvements across all DHI scores and HIT-6 ($p < 0.01$) in addition to the reduction in dizziness and headache frequency. The authors also reported that the home-based VR was adapted from a previous VR programme carried out in adult patients with VM [30].

5.1.2.6 Pathomechanism of VRT's Role in VM

Among the most notable postulations is the link between vestibular and pain pathways in the brain [41, 42] due to the neurochemical similarity found in serotonin and purinergic receptors between vestibular and pain pathway neurons. There is touting evidence that dizziness in VM is associated with ischemia in the central vestibular pathway, spasms of the labyrinthine artery [43], and neurochemical alteration in the vestibular pathway. VR is believed to relieve headaches and dizziness by improving the function of the vestibule through a compensation mechanism [32].

Reports have shown that VM results in disorientation and dizziness in relation to head and body positions, which suggests a dysfunction in multisensory integration for spatial orientation (input from visual, vestibular and somatosensory). Sports and activities that stimulate spatial perception and coordination, such as dancing, can aid in improving symptoms [44]. Evidence shows that these individuals are less visually dependent and process body perceptual and spatial orientation information better [45].

5.1.2.7 Conclusion

We emphasise close collaboration between the Vestibular physician and the child's physiotherapist to tailor each patient's needs individually. The prophylaxis medication may provide the child confidence to perform physical activity. Based on the level of improvement, the physiotherapist can discuss the child's progress with the physician and whether medication needs to be initiated or adjusted [25].

5.1.3 Cognitive Behavioural Therapy

Cognitive behavioural therapy (CBT) is a form of non-pharmacological intervention that modifies behavioural responses to symptoms through active coping skills [46]. It entails psychological education on the gate control theory of pain, deep diaphragmatic breathing, muscle relaxation, guided imagery, activity pacing, cognitive modification, cognitive modification, problem-solving, and cued relaxation [46–48]. CBT aims to address three domains that are believed to trigger or worsen symptoms: behaviours, emotions, and cognition. By changing the patient's thoughts, interpretations and assumptions, patients are made more aware of how to manage stress, coping, and headaches [49, 50].

Myriad research has shown CBT to be a great modality in improving paediatric migraine [46]. Biofeedback, used parallel to relaxation therapy, provides visual data on psychological alteration, such as decreased heart rate and muscle tension [46, 47]. Evidence of the efficacy of psychological intervention for treating various conditions in children has grown substantially.

Nahmah et al., in their study, found that adolescents with migraine who received eight sessions of CBT demonstrated changes in prefrontal cortical activity (PFC) and amygdala [51], which supports the idea that CBT results in alteration in neural functioning in brain regions responsible for cognitive control, emotional regulation, and pain modulation [52].

CBT has been shown to significantly reduce headache days and headache intensity in a randomised clinical trial based on a 2018 Cochrane review on psychological therapies for chronic pain in children and adolescents [53]. The review also reiterated that the number of sessions to achieve an additional benefit outcome of at least 50% improvement of symptoms was low (between 2.59 and 3.58 sessions) [53].

The role of CBT in various vestibular conditions has been well-established [54–56]. Children and adolescents with VM have been shown to be susceptible to developing anxiety. The vestibular system and pathways share neural circuits with pathways responsible for emotional processing, including anxiety [57]. Neural pathways responsible for avoidance, conditioned fear, autonomic arousal, and anxiety have been found to converge in areas related to vestibular processing [57]. Additionally, incorporating VR in individuals with vestibular disorder without addressing the underlying anxiety or emotional issues has been reported to be less effective [54].

Numerous research has advocate CBT as an adjunct to VR [54, 56, 58] as patients are able to cope and handle distorted thinking and alter counterproductive behaviour.

5.1.3.1 Conclusion

CBT has been demonstrated to be efficacious when performed alongside other treatments, such as VR, in both adults and children. The true efficacy of CBT as a single treatment in children and adolescents with VM is not known.

5.1.4 Mindfulness-Based Intervention

Mindfulness-based interventions (MBI) encompass psychoeducational modalities which aim to direct attention in a particular way. The inventions aim to bring one's attention and awareness to the present moment without worrying about the past or present [59]. MBI was first introduced in 1979 by Dr. Jon Kabat-Zinn, who introduced a mindfulness meditation training programme known as Mindfulness-based stress reduction (MBSR), a systematic, intensive training in mindfulness meditation and mindful hatha yoga [60], which demonstrated tremendous success, has ever since been adapted and modified to suit various demographic, gender and population.

MBI has been shown to improve physical health conditions and cognitive, psychosocial, and affective outcomes in adults and children [59, 61, 62].

Over the past decade, tremendous efforts have been made to accommodate MBI children and adolescents. Although some authors have voiced their scepticism about the efficacy of MBI and hold reservations about the metacognitive abilities of children who can benefit from it, recent meta-analyses have proven otherwise [59, 63].

MB I's effectiveness, especially in the domain of symptom reduction and psychological well-being [64], led to it being a part of treatment in many chronic conditions, including migraine [65].

Although no studies on the effect of MBI in children with VM are available yet, MBI has shown promising results among adolescents with headaches [65, 66].

A pilot study by Sansone et al. that incorporated seven sessions of expert-led group-based guided-mindfulness-based meditation of weekly frequency of 45 min, along with home-based practice sessions of 10 minutes, revealed feasibility and sustainability of MBI among adolescents with good outcomes [67]. In another study by Grazzi et al., involving adolescents aged between 12 and 18 with chronic migraine without aura who underwent a seven-week group-based mindfulness meditation without pharmacological prophylaxis demonstrated significant improvement in headache frequency from 21.3 to 9.6 days per month at 12 months ($F = 30.5$, $p < 0.001$) with greater than 50% reduction of headache frequency in 65.7% of participants [66].

functional MRI (fMRI) revealed how cerebral patterns involved in migraine pain are changed through mindfulness, in particular by influencing patterns in the insular region of the cortex [68]. It is worth noting that the insula, a region of the cortex, is responsible for processing and regulating complex sensory and emotional aspects associated with migraine [66].

While the efficacy of MBI among children and adolescents with VM is still being explored, the emerging reports are encouraging. They point towards the potential for more satisfactory and long-term benefits, offering hope for the future of migraine management in younger populations.

5.1.5 Non-invasive Brain Stimulation (NIBS)

NIBS entails neurophysiological intervention involving the transcranial application of electric currents or magnetic fields to modulate brain activity [69]. NIBS has been used for decades to investigate, diagnose, and treat several neuropsychiatric diseases [70].

The first reported application of NIBS goes back to the first century AD by Scribonius Largus, who used a bioelectric fish-black torpedo to deliver an electric pulse to painful areas [71]. The types of NIBS associated with paediatric migraine include transcranial magnetic stimulation (TMS) and transcranial direct current stimulation (tDCS).

Although evidence of NIBS in preventing migraine in the paediatric population is still lacking, some authors have reported promising results. NIBS regulates neuronal excitability and has an excitatory and inhibitory effect, which results in neuromodulation that can alter the activity of several brain connections [69].

Neuromodulation can modify the activity of several brain networks by modulating neuronal excitability and excitatory or inhibitory effects, depending on different stimulation parameters (polarity, duration, or frequency of stimuli). The NIBS techniques have the relevant advantage of inducing brain changes by non-invasive stimulation, which does not require intervention for the application of permanent leads, is painless and optimally tolerated, and can be employed in awake subjects at rest or during the execution of different tasks. These techniques function through transcranial application of magnetic or electric currents (transcranial magnetic [TMS] and electrical stimulation [tES], respectively).

5.1.5.1 Transcranial Magnetic Stimulation

The safety and tolerability of TMS in adults are well-established [72]. Yet, studies on TMS application in children and adolescents remain scarce.

It is worth noting that the magnetic strengths generated by TMS devices are comparable to those of MRI scanners used in clinical practice [73]. Akin to that, noise generated as a result of single-pulse TMS is reported to be 100–120 dB. TMS has been demonstrated to be a safe, effective NPI for migraine in children and adolescents [73]. A prospective pilot study among adolescents between the ages of 12 and 17 for migraine prevention using single-pulse TMS (sTMS) showed good compliance, well-tolerated and acceptable preventative NPI [73]. In an earlier study involving 850 infants and children with neurologic disorders exposed to sTMS, no complications were reported [74].

References

1. Castellano-Tejedor C. Non-pharmacological interventions for the management of chronic health conditions and non-communicable diseases. Int J Environ Res Public Health. 2022;19(14):8536.
2. Neuhauser H, Lempert T. Vestibular migraine. Neurol Clin. 2009;27(2):379–91. https://doi.org/10.1016/j.ncl.2008.11.004.
3. Law EF, et al. Economic impact of headache and psychiatric comorbidities on healthcare expenditures among children in the United States: a retrospective cross-sectional study. Headache. 2019;59(9):1504–15. https://doi.org/10.1111/head.13639.
4. Powers SW, et al. Prevalence of headache days and disability 3 years after participation in the childhood and adolescent migraine prevention medication trial. JAMA Netw Open. 2021;4(7):e2114712.
5. Raucci U, Boni A, Evangelisti M, Della Vecchia N, Velardi M, Ursitti F, Terrin G, Di Nardo G, Reale A, Villani A, Parisi P. Lifestyle modifications to help prevent headache at a developmental age. Front Neurol. 2021;11:618375. https://doi.org/10.3389/fneur.2020.618375. PMID: 33603708; PMCID: PMC7884344
6. Powers SW, Coffey CS, Chamberlin LA, Ecklund DJ, Klingner EA, Yankey JW, et al. Trial of amitriptyline, topiramate, and placebo for pediatric migraine. N Engl J Med. 2017;376:115–24. https://doi.org/10.1056/NEJMoa1610384.
7. Milde-Busch A, Blaschek A, Borggräfe I, Heinen F, Straube A, von Kries R. Associations of diet and lifestyle with headache in high-school students: results from a cross-sectional study. Headache. 2010;50:1104–14. https://doi.org/10.1111/j.1526-4610.2010.01706.x.
8. Martin VT, Vij B. Diet and headache: part 2. Headache. 2016;56:1553–62.
9. Stang PE, Yanagihara PA, Swanson JW, et al. Incidence of migraine headache: a population-based study in Olmsted County, Minnesota. Neurology. 1992;42(9):1657–62. https://doi.org/10.1212/wnl.42.9.1657.
10. Van den Eeden SK, Koepsell TD, Longstreth WT Jr, van Belle G, Daling JR, McKnight B. Aspartame ingestion and headaches: a randomized crossover trial. Neurology. 1994;44(10):1787–93. https://doi.org/10.1212/wnl.44.10.1787.
11. Dalton K, Dalton ME. Food intake before migraine attacks in children. J R Coll Gen Pract. 1979;29(208):662–5. PMID: 544807; PMCID: PMC2159084

12. Neut D, Fily A, Cuvellier JC, Vallée L. The prevalence of triggers in paediatric migraine: a questionnaire study in 102 children and adolescents. J Headache Pain. 2012;13(1):61–5. https://doi.org/10.1007/s10194-011-0397-2. Epub 2011 Nov 1. PMID: 22042255; PMCID: PMC3253155
13. Millichap J, Yee M. The diet factor in paediatric and adolescent migraine. Pediatr Neurol. 2003;28:9–15. https://doi.org/10.1016/S0887-8994(02)00466-6.
14. Reploeg MD, Goebel JA. Migraine-associated dizziness: patient characteristics and management options. Otol Neurotol. 2002;23:364–71.
15. Maione A. Migraine-related vertigo: diagnostic criteria and prophylactic treatment. Laryngoscope. 2006;116:1782–6.
16. Mikulec AA, Faraji F, Kinsella LJ. Evaluation of the efficacy of caffeine cessation, nortriptyline, and topiramate therapy in vestibular migraine and complex dizziness of unknown etiology. Am J Otolaryngol. 2012;33:121–7.
17. Barbanti P, Fofi L, Aurilia C, Egeo G, Caprio M. Ketogenic diet in migraine: rationale, findings and perspectives. Neurol Sci. 2017;38(Suppl. 1):111–5.
18. Herdman SJ, Hall CD, Schubert MC, Das VE, Tusa RJ. Recovery of dynamic visual acuity in bilateral vestibular hypofunction. Arch Otolaryngol Head Neck Surg. 2007;133(4):383–9. https://doi.org/10.1001/archotol.133.4.383.
19. Garcia AP, Gananca MM, Cusin FS, Tomaz A, Gananca FF, Caovilla HH. Vestibular rehabilitation with virtual reality in Meniere's disease. Braz J Otorhinolaryngol. 2013;79:366–74.
20. Webster KE, Galbraith K, Harrington-Benton NA, Judd O, Kaski D, Maarsingh OR, MacKeith S, Ray J, Van Vugt VA, Burton MJ. Non-pharmacological interventions for prophylaxis of vestibular migraine. Cochrane Database Syst Rev. 2023;4:CD015321.
21. Sahin E, Dinc ME, Ozker BY, Cöpürgensli C, Konaklıoglu M, Ozcelik T. The value of vestibular rehabilitation in patients with bilateral vestibular dysfunction. J Int Adv Otol. 2017;13:385–9.
22. Cass SP, Furman JM, Ankerstjerne JK, Balaban C, Yetiser S, Aydogan B. Migraine-related vestibulopathy. Ann Otol Rhinol Laryngol. 1997;106:182–9.
23. Wrisley DM, Whitney SL, Furman JM. Vestibular rehabilitation outcomes in patients with a history of migraine. Otol Neurotol. 2002;23:483–7. https://doi.org/10.1097/00129492-200207000-00016.
24. Suarez H, Arocena M, Suarez A, De Artagaveytia TA, Muse P, Gil J. Changes in postural control parameters after vestibular rehabilitation in patients with central vestibular disorders. Acta Otolaryngol. 2003;123:143–7. https://doi.org/10.1080/0036554021000028109.
25. Whitney SL, Wrisley DM, Brown KE, Furman JM. Physical therapy for migraine-related vestibulopathy and vestibular dysfunction with history of migraine. Laryngoscope. 2000;110:1528–34. https://doi.org/10.1097/00005537-200009000-00022.
26. Brown KE, Whitney SL, Marchetti GF, Wrisley DM, Furman JM. Physical therapy for central vestibular dysfunction. Arch Phys Med Rehabil. 2006;87:76–81. https://doi.org/10.1016/j.apmr.2005.08.003.
27. Johnson GD. Medical management of migraine-related dizziness and vertigo. Laryngoscope. 1988;108(Suppl 85):1–28.
28. Cohen HS, Kimball KT. Increased independence and decreased vertigo after vestibular rehabilitation. Otolaryngol Head Neck Surg. 2003;128:60–70. https://doi.org/10.1067/mhn.2003.23.
29. Gottshall KR, Moore RJ, Hoffer ME. Vestibular rehabilitation for migraine-associated dizziness. Int Tinnitus J. 2005;11(1):81–4.
30. Sugaya N, Arai M, Goto F. Is the headache in patients with vestibular migraine attenuated by vestibular rehabilitation? Front Neurol. 2017;8:124.
31. Koc A, Cevizci Akkılıc E. Effects of vestibular rehabilitation in the management of patients with and without vestibular migraine. Braz J Otorhinolaryngol. 2022;88(Suppl 3):S25–33. https://doi.org/10.1016/j.bjorl.2021.07.011. Epub 2021 Oct 25. PMID: 34799267; PMCID: PMC9760977
32. Shaabani M, Shahrokhi A, Soufinia B, Javanbakht M, Bakhshi E. The effect of vestibular rehabilitation on dizziness and headache in patients with vestibular migraine. Aud Vestib Res. 2019;28(2):87–92.

33. Hall CD, Herdman SJ, Whitney SL, Cass SP, Clendaniel RA, Fife TD, et al. Vestibular rehabilitation for peripheral vestibular hypofunction: an evidence-based clinical practice guideline: from the american physical therapy association neurology section. J Neurol Phys Ther. 2016;40:124–55. https://doi.org/10.1097/NPT.0000000000000120.
34. Rine RM. Vestibular rehabilitation for children. Semin Hear. 2018;39(3):334–44.
35. Lacour M, Bernard-Demanze L. Interaction between vestibular compensation mechanisms and vestibular rehabilitation therapy: 10 recommendations for optimal functional recovery. Front Neurol. 2015;5(285):285.
36. Bisdorff AR. Management of vestibular migraine. Ther Adv Neurol Disord. 2011;4:183–91. https://doi.org/10.1177/1756285611401647.
37. Furman JM, Balaban CD, Jacob RG, Marcus DA. Migraine-anxiety related dizziness (MARD): a new disorder? J Neurol Neurosurg Psychiatry. 2005;76:1–8. https://doi.org/10.1136/jnnp.2004.048926.
38. Power L, Shute W, McOwan B, Murray K, Szmulewicz D. Clinical characteristics and treatment choice in vestibular migraine. J Clin Neurosci. 2018;52:50–3. https://doi.org/10.1016/j.jocn.2018.02.020.
39. Jacob RG, Woody SR, Duncan DB, et al. Discomfort with space and motion: a possible marker for vestibular dysfunction assessed by a situational characteristics questionnaire. J Psychopathol Behav Assess. 1994;15:299–324.
40. Vitkovic J, Winoto A, Rance G, Dowell R, Paine M. Vestibular rehabilitation outcomes in patients with and without vestibular migraine. J Neurol. 2013;260(12):3039–48. https://doi.org/10.1007/s00415-013-7116-7.
41. Ohno K, Takeda N, Yamano M, Matsunaga T, Tohyama M. Coexistence of acetylcholine and calcitonin gene-related peptide in the vestibular efferent neurons in the rat. Brain Res. 1991;566(1-2):103–7. https://doi.org/10.1016/0006-8993(91)91686-U.
42. Lewis RF, Priesol AJ, Nicoucar K, Lim K, Merfeld DM. Abnormal motion perception in vestibular migraine. Laryngoscope. 2011;121(5):1124–5. https://doi.org/10.1002/lary.2172.
43. Pérez PD, Beltrán MLD, del Cañizo AA, Sancipriano JA, Calvo BE, Benito GJJ. Benign paroxysmal vertigo in childhood. Acta Otorrinolaringol Esp. 1998;49(2):151–5.
44. Huang TC, Wang SJ, Kheradmand A. Vestibular migraine: an update on current understanding and future directions. Cephalalgia. 2020;40(1):107–21. https://doi.org/10.1177/0333102419869317. Epub 2019 Aug 8
45. Fiori F, David N, Aglioti SM. Processing of proprioceptive and vestibular body signals and self-transcendence in Ashtanga yoga practitioners. Front Hum Neurosci. 2014;8(734):174.
46. Eccleston C, Fisher E, Law E, Bartlett J, Palermo TM. Psychological interventions for parents of children and adolescents with chronic illness. Cochrane Database Syst Rev. 2015;4:CD009660.
47. Powers SW, Kashikar-Zuck SM, Allen JR, LeCates SL, Slater SK, Zafar M, Kabbouche MA, O'Brien HL, Shenk CE, Rausch JR, Hershey AD. Cognitive behavioral therapy plus amitriptyline for chronic migraine in children and adolescents: a randomized clinical trial. JAMA. 2013;310:2622–30.
48. Kroon Van Diest AM, Ernst MM, Vaughn L, Slater S, Powers SW. CBT for Pediatric Migraine: A Qualitative Study of Patient and Parent Experience. Headache. 2018;58(5):661–675.
49. Rains JC, Penzien DB, McCrory DC, Gray RN. Behavioral headache treatment: history, review of the empirical literature, and methodological critique. Headache. 2005;45(s2):S92–S109.
50. Kabbouche MA, Gilman DK. Management of migraine in adolescents. Neuropsychiatr Dis Treat. 2008;4(3):535–48.
51. Nahman-Averbuch H, et al. Alterations in brain function after cognitive behavioral therapy for migraine in children and adolescents. Headache. 2020;60(6):1165–82.
52. Knestrick KE, Gibler RC, Reidy BL, Powers SW. Psychological interventions for pediatric headache disorders: a 2021 update on research progress and needs. Curr Pain Headache Rep. 2022;26(1):85–91. https://doi.org/10.1007/s11916-022-01007-z. Epub 2022 Feb 2. PMID: 35107711; PMCID: PMC8807374

53. Fisher E, et al. Psychological therapies for the management of chronic and recurrent pain in children and adolescents. Cochrane Database Syst Rev. 2018;9(9):Cd003968.
54. Naber CM, Water-Schmeder O, Bohrer PS, Matonak K, Bernstein AL, Merchant MA. Interdisciplinary treatment for vestibular dysfunction: the effectiveness of mindfulness, cognitive-behavioral techniques, and vestibular rehabilitation. Otolaryngol Head Neck Surg. 2011;145(1):117–24.
55. Kristiansen L, Magnussen LH, Wilhelmsen KT, et al. Efficacy of intergrating vestibular rehabilitation and cognitive behaviour therapy in persons with persistent dizziness in primary care—a study protocol for a randomised controlled trial. Trials. 2019;20(1):575. Published 2019 Oct 7. https://doi.org/10.1186/s13063-019-3660-5.
56. Kristiansen L, Magnussen LH, Juul-Kristensen B, et al. Feasibility of integrating vestibular rehabilitation and cognitive behaviour therapy for people with persistent dizziness. Pilot Feasibility Stud. 2019;5:69. Published 2019 May 20. https://doi.org/10.1186/s40814-019-0452-3.
57. Balaban C, Thayer JF. Neurological bases for balance-anxiety links. J Anxiety Disord. 2001;15:53–79.
58. Beidel DC, Horak FB. Behavior therapy for vestibular rehabilitation. J Anxiety Disord. 2001;15:121–30.
59. Lin J, Chadi N, Shrier L. Mindfulness-based interventions for adolescent health. Curr Opin Pediatr. 2019;31(4):469–75. https://doi.org/10.1097/MOP.0000000000000760. PMID: 30939515
60. Kabat-Zinn J. An outpatient program in behavioral medicine for chronic pain patients based on the practice of mindfulness meditation: theoretical considerations and preliminary results. Gen Hosp Psychiatry. 1982;4(1):33–47.
61. Dunning DL, Griffiths K, Kuyken W, Crane C, Foulkes L, Parker J, et al. Research review: the effects of mindfulness-based interventions on cognition and mental health in children and adolescents—a meta-analysis of randomized controlled trials. J Child Psychol Psychiatr. 2019;60(3):244–58.
62. Zoogman S, Goldberg SB, Hoyt WT, Miller L. Mindfulness interventions with youth: a meta-analysis. Mindfulness. 2015;6(2):290–302.
63. Mettler J, Khoury B, Zito S, Sadowski I, Heath NL. Mindfulness-based programs and school adjustment: a systematic review and meta-analysis. J Sch Psychol. 2023;97:43–62. https://doi.org/10.1016/j.jsp.2022.10.007. Epub 2023 Jan 25
64. Choudhury S, Moses JM. Mindful interventions: youth, poverty, and the developing brain. Theory Psychol. 2016;26:591–606.
65. Hesse T, Holmes LG, Kennedy-Overfelt V, Kerr LM, Giles LL. Mindfulness-based intervention for adolescents with recurrent headaches: a pilot feasibility study. Evid Based Complement Alternat Med. 2015;2015:508958. https://doi.org/10.1155/2015/508958. Epub 2015 Dec 22. PMID: 26798398; PMCID: PMC4700163
66. Grazzi L, Grignani E, Raggi A, Rizzoli P, Guastafierro E. Effect of a mindfulness-based intervention for chronic migraine and high frequency episodic migraine in adolescents: a pilot single-arm open-label study. Int J Environ Res Public Health. 2021;18(22):11739. https://doi.org/10.3390/ijerph182211739. PMID: 34831494; PMCID: PMC8619568
67. Sansone E, Raggi A, Grignani E, Leonardi M, D'Amico D, Scaratti C, Grazzi L. Mindfulness meditation for chronic migraine in pediatric population: a pilot study. Neurol Sci. 2018;39(Suppl 1):111–3. https://doi.org/10.1007/s10072-018-3365-7.
68. Borsook D, Veggeberg R, Erpelding N, Borra R, Linnman C, Burstein R, Becerra L. The insula: a "hub of activity" in migraine. Neuroscientist. 2016;22(6):632–52. https://doi.org/10.1177/1073858415601369. Epub 2015 Aug 19. PMID: 26290446; PMCID: PMC5723020
69. Brighina F, Raieli V, Messina LM, Santangelo G, Puma D, Drago F, Rocchitelli L, Vanadia F, Giglia G, Mangano S. Non-invasive brain stimulation in pediatric migraine: a perspective from evidence in adult migraine. Front Neurol. 2019;10:364. https://doi.org/10.3389/fneur.2019.00364. PMID: 31031695; PMCID: PMC6473052

70. Jenkins B, Tepper SJ. Neurostimulation for primary headache disorders, part 1, pathophysiology and anatomy, history of neuromodulation in headache treatment, and review of peripheral neuromodulation in primary headaches. Headache. 2011;51:1254–66. https://doi.org/10.1111/j.1526-4610.2011.01966.x.
71. Wagner T, Valero-Cabre A, Pascual-Leone A. A brief summary of the history of noninvasive brain stimulation. Annu Rev Biomed Eng. 2007;9:527–65. https://doi.org/10.1146/annurev.bioeng.9.061206.133100.
72. Zewdie E, Ciechanski P, Kuo HC, et al. Safety and tolerability of transcranial magnetic and direct current stimulation in children: prospective single center evidence from 3.5 million stimulations. Brain Stimul. 2020;13(3):565–75. https://doi.org/10.1016/j.brs.2019.12.025.
73. Irwin SL, Qubty W, Allen IE, Patniyot I, Goadsby PJ, Gelfand AA. Transcranial magnetic stimulation for migraine prevention in adolescents: a pilot open-label study. Headache. 2018;58(5):724–31. https://doi.org/10.1111/head.13284. Epub 2018 Mar 12. PMID: 29528485
74. Gilbert DL, Garvey MA, Bansal AS, Lipps T, Zhang J, Wassermann EM. Should transcranial magnetic stimulation research in children be considered minimal risk? Clin Neurophysiol. 2004;115:1730–9.

Vestibular Migraine in Adolescent: How it Differs from Children

6

Jeyasakthy Saniasiaya, Jeyanthi Kulasegarah, and Narayanan Prepageran

6.1 Introduction

Adolescence comes from the Latin word *adolescere*, which means to grow, to mature [1]. Adolescence can be termed as a period from the onset of puberty till early adulthood [2]. More than half a decade ago, the World Health Organization [3] proposed that adolescence is a period between 10 to 20 years, although the endpoint of the adolescence period was less defined [4, 5]. It was when the United Nations (UN) Convention on the Rights of the Child defined a child as an individual aged between 0 and 18; adolescence was formally defined as the period between 10 and 19 years of age [6]. Having said that, we must acknowledge that adolescence's defining age may vary across cultures and countries worldwide.

Regardless of age, we all must agree that adolescence is a critical period in an individual's life. It is a period in which a child transitions into adulthood. It is also an essential period of development concerning biological, physical, psychosocial, and emotional changes.

Historically, vestibular conditions among adolescents have been assumed to be similar to those of children (under 10 years of age). Adolescents possess the characteristics of both a child and an adult, making their management challenging [7].

J. Saniasiaya (✉) · J. Kulasegarah · N. Prepageran
Department of Otorhinolaryngology, Faculty of Medicine, Universiti Malaya, Kuala Lumpur, Wilayah Persekutuan Kuala Lumpur, Malaysia
e-mail: jeyasakthy@um.edu.my

J. Saniasiaya (ed.), *Vestibular Migraine in Children and Adolescents: An overview*, https://doi.org/10.1007/978-981-96-2167-5_6

6.2 Physiological Changes in Adolescents

Several major cortical pathways involved in executive, attention, and regulatory functions continue to develop during adolescence period [8]. The vestibular system matures approximately at the age of 16 [9]. The functional development of the vestibular system alters an adolescent's somatosensory and visual control of postural control [9]. In addition to the ongoing changes that occur to the vestibular system, external factors such as asthenic habitus, increased stress, poor and sedentary lifestyle, substance abuse, sleep deprivation, and hormonal changes with increased migraine rates alter the somatosensorial control resulting in vertigo or dizziness among adolescents [10].

6.3 Incidence of Vestibular Migraine among Adolescents

The incidence of dizziness or vertigo in adolescents has increased over the past decade. Five to ten per cent of adolescents reported having at least one episode of vertigo [11]. Approximately 18% of adolescents were reported to have one episode of vertigo by age 15, while 5.3% had more frequent vertigo episodes [12, 13]. Adolescents between 11 and 15 years old have been demonstrated to experience vertigo with a peak at 12 [12]. The exact incidence of VM among adolescents remains unknown until a large-scale, multicenter study using standardized criteria for VM is conducted.

6.4 Risk Factors

6.4.1 Gender and Hormonal Influence

Female adolescents are more susceptible to VM than males. Wang et al. reported that female adolescents are found to be more prone to develop multiple concurrent vestibular disorders than their male counterparts [14], which has been linked to hormonal factors [15, 16].

Studies have shown that both endogen and exogen estrogens can alter vestibular function [17]. Estrogen receptors were reported to be found at the stria vascularis and spiral ligament [17]. Hormonal changes during puberty and the menstrual cycle can alter or cause estrogen fluctuations, subsequently altering the homeostasis of labyrinthine fluids and directly influencing the enzymatic process and neurotransmitter function [18]. Variations of the labyrinthine fluid's homeostasis and alteration of the sensitivity on the enzymatic receptors are postulated to cause vestibular symptoms in female adolescents [17].

6.4.2 BPVC

Reports that children with benign paroxysmal vertigo of childhood lead to adult migraine have been well established. It is worth noting that children who were earlier diagnosed with benign paroxysmal vertigo of childhood are prone to develop VM during the adolescent period [19].

6.4.3 Poor Lifestyle

New emerging evidence of risk factors resulting from lifestyle affecting VM in adolescents includes stress, poor sleep, alcohol and recreational drugs, smoking, including e-cigarettes and a poor sedentary lifestyle.

6.4.4 Role of Epigenetics

VM is a dynamic condition. The role of epigenetics among migraineurs has recently emerged [20]. Epigenetics involves the phenotypic alteration resulting from modified genetic expression [21]. Understanding the pathomechanism and impact of epigenetic alteration on VM, especially among adolescents, would enable a better understanding of risk factors, pathogenesis, disease progression and outcome of VM and aid targeted or individualized treatment. Epigenetics study on VM in both children and adolescents. Research has shown that epigenetic alteration in adolescents with VM can be passed on from generation to generation [22] and influence embryonic and postnatal development [23].

6.5 How Vestibular Migraine Differs in Adolescents

Neuroplasticity, which enables better tolerability to vertigo, resulting in a short-lived duration of symptoms and self-limiting symptoms, is reduced in adolescents [19].

Vestibular assessments used to assess children are unsuitable for adolescents, and assessments performed in adults may be too strenuous for adolescents. Criteria and assessments must be tailored to the adolescent age group; however, adolescents are pooled along with younger children.

Regarding presentation, adolescents present with bilateral headaches compared to adults [24].

Overlap between two or more vestibular diagnoses has been mentioned in the literature since the early twentieth century [25]. Reports on the multifactorial contributing vestibular diagnosis in a single patient have been known among adult patients [26–28]. Approximately, 3.7% of the population is estimated to receive two or more vestibular diagnoses concurrently, although the true incidence may be higher [29–31]. In the adult population, VM has been frequently reported to be found concurrently with other vestibular conditions, especially BPPV, MD, bilateral vestibulopathy, PPPD, and somatoform vertigo [26]. While the exact mechanism of each vestibular condition remains not fully understood, myriad research has been ongoing to explore the relationship between these conditions. It is worth noting that the robust and extensive connections between the vestibular system and various parts of the brain and other sensory systems explain the multitude of vestibular diagnoses in a single individual.

Recent reports on multifactorial contributing factors of vestibular conditions among adolescents have emerged. Therefore, a single adolescent can have two or more vestibular conditions that must be addressed, which leads to the complexity of managing the affected adolescent. In a study by Wang et al., that aimed to identify multifactorial characteristics of pediatric dizziness, 44.4% of the included children (mean 12.5 ± 4.9 years) were found to have multiple contributing diagnoses whereby children with VM were found to be diagnosed with BPPV or PPPD. Interestingly, in their study, 22 children were diagnosed with VM, BBPV and PPPD [14]. Although the exact pathomechanism of VM and BPPV remains elusive, it has been postulated that utricular impairment and otoconial displacement occur secondary to inflammatory changes in the inner ear [32]. As for PPPD and VM, prior vestibular disorders, notably BPPV and PPPD, have been demonstrated to occur concurrently or precipitate PPPD in adolescents [33].

Motion sickness has been identified to occur concomitantly with VM in adolescents, which may pose a challenge in management. Disturbance in the visual system, spatial orientation, and the inability to integrate multisensory input has been shown to cause a visual-vestibular conflict [18].

Failure to identify multifactorial contributing diagnoses could delay recovery and result in long-term consequences from a vestibular impairment, including cognition, balance and posture, and psychosocial and emotional disturbance.

6.5.1 Chronicity of VM in Adolescents

Research and studies on VM in adolescents, which remain scarce, lead to a poor understanding of the pathomechanism of the progression of VM in the adolescent period.

We are unsure of the disease progression of children diagnosed with VM early in childhood in the adolescent period. Adolescents with migraines may have dizziness components that may have been underlooked or under-recognized, resulting in a lower incidence. Reports have shown that chronic migraine is associated with trouble sleeping, dizziness, anxiety and mood, muscle pain, and abdominal conditions [34].

Adolescents may suffer from a more chronic type of symptoms with periods of headache and dizziness that may alternate or present concurrently.

6.6 Conclusion

Adolescents are in a critical period of life, transitioning from being a child into being an adult. While processing the physical, emotional and psychosocial changes during puberty, understanding and processing their symptoms may pose a challenge. It is important to be aware that VM in adolescents can occur as a stand-alone condition or concurrent with another vestibular condition, notably BPPV and PPPD. Physicians must be aware that adolescents are not children and that their approach to vestibular conditions needs to be tailored accordingly. Concurrent vestibular disorders that can occur along with VM must be investigated thoroughly.

References

1. Sawyer SM, Azzopardi PS, Wickremarathne D, Patton GC. The age of adolescence. Lancet Child Adolesc Health. 2018;2(3):223–8.
2. National Academies of Sciences, Engineering, and Medicine, Health and Medicine Division, Division of Behavioral and Social Sciences and Education, Board on Children, Youth, and Families, Committee on the Neurobiological and Socio-behavioral Science of Adolescent Development and Its Applications. In: Backes EP, Bonnie RJ, editors. The promise of adolescence: realizing opportunity for all youth. Washington, DC: National Academies Press (US); 2019.
3. WHO. The global strategy for women's, children's, and adolescents' health (2016–30). 2015. http://www.who.int/life-course/partners/global-strategy/ewec-globalstrategyreport-200915.pdf?ua=1. Accessed 30 Mar 2024.
4. WHO. Health problems of adolescents. Technical report series 308. Geneva: World Health Organization; 1965.
5. WHO. Health needs of adolescents. Geneva: World Health Organization; 1977.
6. United Nations Children's Fund, UNICEF Programme Guidance for the Second Decade: Programming with and for Adolescents, Programme Division, UNICEF, October 2018:9.
7. Lee JD, Kim CH, Hong SM, et al. Prevalence of vestibular and balance disorders in children and adolescents according to age: a multi-center study. Int J Pediatr Otorhinolaryngol. 2017;94:36–9.
8. Toga AW, Thompson PM, Sowell ER. Mapping brain maturation. Trends Neurosci. 2006;29:148–59. https://doi.org/10.1016/j.tins.2006.01.007.
9. Cumberworth VL, Patel NN, Rogers W, Kenyon GS. The maturation of balance in children. J Laryngol Otol. 2007;121:449–54.
10. Filippopulos FM, Albers L, Straube A, et al. Vertigo and dizziness in adolescents: risk factors and their population attributable risk. PLoS One. 2017;12(11):e0187819.
11. Deissler A, Albers L, von Kries R, et al. Health-related quality of life of children/adolescents with vertigo: retrospective study from the German Center of Vertigo and Balance Disorders. Neuropediatrics. 2017;48:91–7.
12. Gioacchini FM, Alicandri-Ciufelli M, Kaleci S, Magliulo G, Re M. Prevalence and diagnosis of vestibular disorders in children: a review. Int J Pediatr Otorhinolaryngol. 2014;78(5):718–24. https://doi.org/10.1016/j.ijporl.2014.02.009.
13. Brodsky JR, Lipson S, Bhattacharyya N. Prevalence of pediatric dizziness and imbalance in the United States. Otolaryngol Head Neck Surg. 2020;162(2):241–7. https://doi.org/10.1177/0194599819887375.
14. Wang A, Zhou G, Lipson S, Kawai K, Corcoran M, Brodsky JR. Multifactorial characteristics of pediatric dizziness and imbalance. Laryngoscope. 2021;131(4):E1308–14.

15. Sacco S, Ricci S, Degan D, Carolei A. Migraine in women: the role of hormones and their impact on vascular diseases. J Headache Pain. 2012;13:177–89.
16. Mattsson P. Hormonal factors in migraine: a population-based study of women aged 40 to 74 years. Headache. 2003;43:27–35.
17. Castillo-Bustamante M, del Cid CC, Vázquez M, Bello Dotel L, Baez Recalde M. Estrogen and neurotological dividers in women sexual hormones and neurotological disorders in women [article in Spanish]. Rev Fac Cien Med Univ Nac Cordoba. 2020;77:351–5.
18. Nocini R, Baraldi C, Apa E, Ciorba A, Monzani D, Palma S. Visually evoked postural responses (VEPRs) in children with vestibular migraine. Children (Basel). 2021;9:14.
19. Saniasiaya J, Narayanan P. Vestibular dysfunction amongst adolescents: what do we know? A review. J Laryngol Otol. 2023;137(1):2–6. https://doi.org/10.1017/S0022215122001268.
20. Zobdeh F, Eremenko II, Akan MA, Tarasov VV, Chubarev VN, Schiöth HB, Mwinyi J. The epigenetics of migraine. Int J Mol Sci. 2023;24(11):9127.
21. Mittal R, Bencie N, Liu G, Eshraghi N, Nisenbaum E, Blanton SH, Yan D, Mittal J, Dinh CT, Young JI, Gong F, Liu XZ. Recent advancements in understanding the role of epigenetics in the auditory system. Gene. 2020;761:144996.
22. National Human Genome Research Institute. Available online: https://www.genome.gov/search?terms=epigenetics Accessed 16 Nov 2023.
23. Balendran V, Ritter KE, Martin DM. Epigenetic mechanisms of inner ear development. Hear Res. 2022;426:108440.
24. Pavlou M, Whitney SL, Alkathiry AA, et al. Visually induced dizziness in children and validation of the pediatric visually induced dizziness questionnaire. Front Neurol. 2017;8:656.
25. Neumann H, Ruttin E. Zur Aetiologie der akuten Otitis. Archiv für Ohrenheilkunde. 1909;79(1-2):1–22.
26. Zhu RT, Van Rompaey V, Ward BK, Van de Berg R, Van de Heyning P, Sharon JD. The interrelations between different causes of dizziness: a conceptual framework for understanding vestibular disorders. Ann Otol Rhinol Laryngol. 2019;128:869–78.
27. Muelleman T, Shew M, Subbarayan R, et al. Epidemiology of dizzy patient population in a Neurotology clinic and predictors of peripheral etiology. Otol Neurotol. 2017;38:870–5.
28. van Leeuwen RB, Colijn C, van Wensen E, Bruintjes TD. The dizzy patient: consider a second diagnosis. Neurologist. 2017;22:69–71.
29. Strupp M, Brandt T, Huppert D, Grill E. Prevalence of motion sickness in various vestibular disorders: a study on 749 patients. J Neurol. 2018;265(suppl 1):95–7.
30. Feil K, Feuerecker R, Goldschagg N, et al. Predictive capability of an iPad-based medical device (medx) for the diagnosis of vertigo and dizziness. Front Neurol. 2018;9:29.
31. Pan Q, Zhang Y, Long T, et al. Diagnosis of vertigo and dizziness syndromes in a neurological outpatient clinic. Eur Neurol. 2018;79(5-6):287–94.
32. Koo JW, Balaban CD. Serotonin-induced plasma extravasation in the murine inner ear: possible mechanism of migraine-associated inner ear dysfunction. Cephalalgia. 2006;26:1310–9.
33. Best C, Tschan R, Eckhardt-Henn A, Dieterich M. Who is at risk for ongoing dizziness and psychological strain after a vestibular disorder? Neuroscience. 2009;164:1579–87.
34. Youssef PE, Mack KJ. Episodic and chronic migraine in children. Dev Med Child Neurol. 2020;62(1):34–41. https://doi.org/10.1111/dmcn.14338.

Conditions Associated with Vestibular Migraine in Pediatric Patients

7

Carolyn M. Jenks and Jacob R. Brodsky

Vestibular migraine is the most common disorder among pediatric patients presenting for the evaluation of dizziness. Migraine variants affect patients throughout the lifespan. Younger patients present with variants including benign paroxysmal torticollis of infancy and recurrent vertigo of childhood, which may predate development of vestibular migraine. Vestibular migraine often co-occurs with other non-migraine diagnoses as well. Studies in children with dizziness report more than one diagnosis in a substantial proportion of patients (44% of children in one large study) [1]. Comorbid conditions impact the treatment and recovery of patients with vestibular migraine and must be recognized and managed concurrently. Overlapping symptoms make diagnosis of multiple concurrent etiologies challenging. This chapter provides an overview of pediatric migraine variants as well as related conditions that occur in pediatric patients with migraine.

7.1 Pediatric Migraine Variants

Pediatric migraine variants share common features including episodic nature, family history of migraine, and progression to migraine. Headache is often absent in pediatric migraine variants, which sometimes makes diagnosis challenging.

C. M. Jenks
Department of Otolaryngology—Head and Neck Surgery, Johns Hopkins University, Baltimore, MD, USA

J. R. Brodsky (✉)
Department of Otolaryngology and Communication Enhancement, Boston Children's Hospital, Harvard Medical School, Boston, MA, USA
e-mail: jacob.brodsky@childrens.harvard.edu

J. Saniasiaya (ed.), *Vestibular Migraine in Children and Adolescents: An overview*, https://doi.org/10.1007/978-981-96-2167-5_7

7.1.1 Benign Paroxysmal Torticollis of Infancy

Benign paroxysmal torticollis of infancy (BPTI) results in intermittent episodes of cervical dystonia (Fig. 7.1). Children may also experience agitation, pallor, nausea, vomiting, gait instability, and/or falls during episodes. Children typically have a normal neurological examination between episodes. Onset of BPTI most often occurs by 7 months of age but may present in the first few years of life [2]. Episodes remit by age 2–3 years in the majority of cases. Gross motor delays have been reported among half or more of patients with BPTI [2, 3]. In children with recurrent acute otitis media, episodes have been reported to flare in the setting of infections [3].

Diagnosis of BPTI is made clinically using criteria from the International Classification of Headache Disorders, third edition (ICHD3; Fig. 7.2) [4]. Treatment is typically unnecessary given the benign and self-limited nature of the condition, though cyproheptadine may be used in severe cases. Children with recurrent acute otitis media and BPTI may benefit from tympanostomy tube placement.

Children with BPTI often develop other migraine variants as they progress into later childhood and adolescence, including recurrent vertigo of childhood (RVC, 43% in one study), cyclical vomiting, and vestibular migraine (aka, the "Vestibular March") [3, 5]. There is often a family history of migraine and sometimes a family history of familial hemiplegic migraine or episodic ataxia [2, 6]. An association has

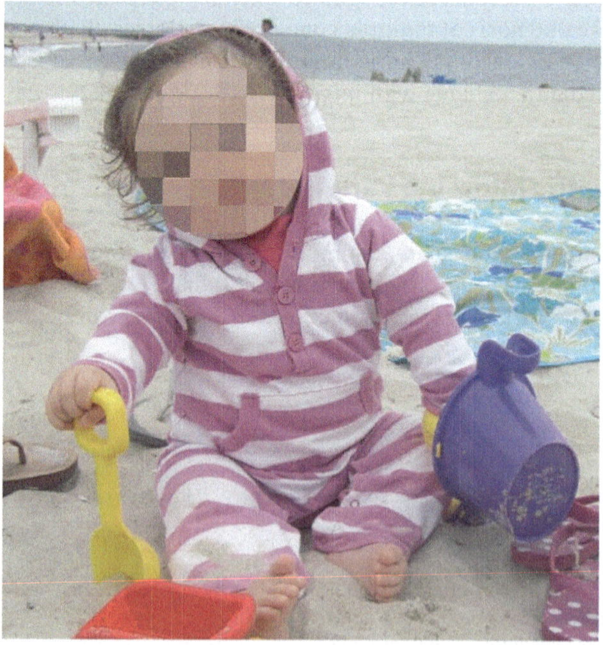

Fig. 7.1 Image of a child during a benign paroxysmal torticollis of infancy flare. Reprinted with permission from Brodsky et al. 2018 [3]

A. Recurrent attacks in infants and small children
B. Head tilt to either side that remits spontaneously after minutes to days
C. At least one of the following symptoms is present: pallor, irritability, malaise, vomiting, ataxia
D. Normal neurological examination between attacks
E. Not attributed to another disorder.

Fig. 7.2 Diagnostic criteria for benign paroxysmal torticollis of infancy (BPTI)

also been reported between BPTI and the CACNA1A genetic mutation that causes episodic ataxia type 2 [6, 7], though it could be argued that such patients may not represent true migrainous BPTI and instead were patients with early onset episodic ataxia, which should be included in the differential diagnosis of children presenting with episodic torticollis symptoms. Paroxysmal torticollis has also been associated with enlarged vestibular aqueducts (EVA), and symptoms of BPTI may precede the development of hearing loss in these children [8]. Because of this association, the authors advocate for annual audiometric testing until at least the age of 5 in children presenting with paroxysmal torticollis, and imaging studies of the temporal bone may be worthwhile if the suspicion for EVA is high, particularly when sensorineural or mixed hearing loss is also present.

7.1.2 Recurrent Vertigo of Childhood

Recurrent vertigo of childhood (RVC), previously known as benign paroxysmal vertigo of childhood (BPVC), is a pediatric migraine variant that most commonly affects young and school-aged children. Typical age of onset is around 3–6 years, but it may present throughout the first decade of life and even occasionally in adolescents [3]. Onset of symptoms is sudden, and symptoms usually last for minutes, but they may last for hours. Vertigo is often severe and causes children to hold onto something or get down on the ground for stability. Diagnostic criteria, defined by the Bárány Society and the International Headache Society are included in Fig. 7.3 [9]. Children with associated migraine symptoms such as nausea, vomiting, photophobia, phonophobia are classified as probable or definite vestibular migraine, though they would have previously been included in the category of BPVC.

Diagnosis is made clinically using the aforementioned diagnostic criteria. Treatment is typically unnecessary given the benign and self-limited nature of the disease. Children with severe and frequent episodes may be treated with cyproheptadine, which is often very effective at preventing symptom flares [3]. Episodes typically become less frequent over time and remit within 2 years of onset, on average (Fig. 7.4) [10].

Although the criteria and clinical presentation of BPVC and RVC, most studies on the natural history of this condition rely on the diagnostic criteria for BPVC, given that the RVC terminology and criteria are relatively new as of the time of this

A. At least three episodes with vestibular symptoms of moderate or severe intensity, lasting between 1 minute and 72 hours
B. None of the criteria B and C for Vestibular Migraine of Childhood**
C. Age < 18 years
D. Not better accounted for by another headache disorder, vestibular disorder, or other condition

Fig. 7.3 Diagnostic criteria for recurrent vertigo of childhood (RVC)*. *Note: The International Classification of Headache Disorders has not been updated since criteria for RVC were established and still uses the term benign paroxysmal vertigo of childhood (BPVC). **Criteria B and C for Vestibular Migraine of Childhood are: (B) A current or past history of migraine with or without aura. (C) At least half of episodes are associated with at least one of the following three migraine features: (1) Headache with at least two of the following four characteristics: (a) One sided location, (b) Pulsating quality, (c) Moderate or severe pain intensity, (d) Aggravation by routine physical activity. (2) Photophobia and phonophobia. (3) Visual aura

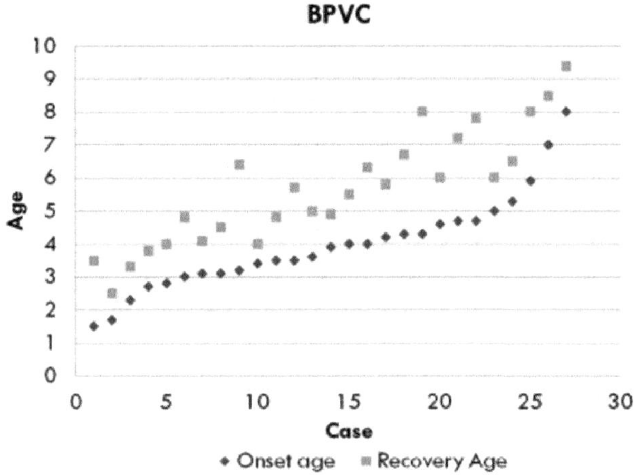

Fig. 7.4 Age of onset and remission of 27 children with benign paroxysmal vertigo of childhood. Reprinted with permission from Batuecas-Caletrío et al. 2013 [10]

writing. Children with BPVC have two times increased risk of developing migraine in adulthood, with 20–69% of children with BPVC later developing migraine [10–13]. In one large series of children with BPVC, 15% of patients developed vestibular migraine later in childhood or adulthood [3].

7.1.3 Cyclical Vomiting

Cyclical vomiting (CVS) is a disorder of gut–brain interaction that results in recurrent episodes of sudden-onset nausea, vomiting, and abdominal pain. Although it has not been shown to have a specific vestibular component to its symptoms or pathophysiology, it is included in this section since the symptoms of episodic

Neonate/Toddler
Must include all of the following:
1. Two or more periods of unremitting paroxysmal vomiting with or without retching, lasting hours to days within a 6-month period
2. Episodes are stereotypical in each patient
3. Episodes are separated by weeks to months with return to baseline health between episodes of vomiting

Child/Adolescent
Must include all of the following:
1. The occurrence of 2 or more periods of intense, unremitting nausea and paroxysmal vomiting, lasting hours to days within a 6-month period.
2. Episodes are stereotypical in each patient
3. Episodes are separated by weeks to months with return to baseline health between episodes.
4. After appropriate medical evaluation, the symptoms cannot be attributed to another condition.

Fig. 7.5 Cyclic vomiting syndrome diagnostic criteria [16, 17]

nausea and vomiting are often also associated with vestibular disorders, including vestibular migraine and its variants. It affects both children and adults, though the average age of onset in childhood is 5 years with a female predominance [14]. Patients may also experience pallor and lethargy. Episodes typically last 2–3 days with most severe symptoms present the onset [15]. Between episodes, patients have minimal or no symptoms. Symptom onset often occurs overnight or in the early morning. The pathophysiology is complex, involving genetic, neuroendocrine, and cognitive/behavioral factors, and it is believed to be a migraine variant, with many patients also affected by other forms of migraine and having a family history of migraine. Similar to other forms of migraine, there are often identifiable triggers including weather changes, illness, poor sleep, motion sickness, menstruation, and stress.

Diagnosis of CVS is made clinically after excluding other diagnoses. Clinical criteria have been adapted from the Rome IV criteria for infants and toddlers as well as children and adolescents (Fig. 7.5) [16–18]. Workup typically involves upper endoscopy and imaging studies. Treatment involves avoidance of triggers, supportive care during episodes, migraine prophylactic agents (antidepressants, antiepileptics), abortive agents (anti-emetics, triptans) as well as management of comorbid anxiety and depression, when present.

7.2 Vestibular Conditions Associated with Migraine

The following conditions can either occur concurrently with vestibular migraine or may be confused with vestibular migraine and should be considered when diagnosing a patient with episodic vertigo symptoms.

7.2.1 Benign Paroxysmal Positional Vertigo

Benign paroxysmal positional vertigo (BPPV) is caused by the displacement of otoconia crystals from the utricle into one or more of the semicircular canals (canalithiasis) or onto one of the semicircular canal cupulae (cupulolithiasis). Patients typically report discrete episodes of vertigo with head movements such as rolling over in bed or looking up or down. Vertigo typically lasts for seconds to minutes. Though true spinning vertigo is most commonly reported, patients sometimes report light headedness, dizziness, nausea, or dysequilibrium. The posterior canal is most commonly affected in both children and adults and accounts for 85–95% of cases in adults, however, horizontal, superior, and multi-canal involvement have all been reported more commonly in children compared with adults [19].

BPPV is usually idiopathic in adults and is thought to be related to age-related degeneration of the utricle organ, but in children, it occurs most often as a result of head trauma. In one large series, it caused about a third of persistent dizziness after concussion [19]. BPPV is diagnosed in 1–5% of children being seen for dizziness, though rates are higher in studies with an increased proportion of post-concussive patients [20–23]. BPPV occurs more commonly among adolescents and females.

Diagnosis of BPPV is performed with head positioning maneuvers specific to each canal, which elicit dizziness and nystagmus [24, 25]. Nystagmus with each of these maneuvers typically has a latency of 5–20 s and fatigues within 60 s. Posterior canal BPPV is diagnosed by the Dix Hallpike maneuver. The patient's head is turned 45° to one side and they are rapidly moved from seated to supine with head hanging at about 20°. This will result in a brief episode of vertigo and upbeating, geotropic torsional (eyes rotating toward the floor) nystagmus in patients with posterior semicircular canal BPPV on the side facing toward the floor.

The supine head roll maneuver is used to diagnose BPPV of the horizontal semicircular canals. The patient lays in the supine position on the exam table with head flexed at about 30°. The head is then rotated approximately 90° to the side by the examiner. A positive test elicits vertigo and horizontal nystagmus, the direction of which is theorized to depend on whether the otoconia crystals are located in the long arm of the semicircular canal (canalithiasis) or adherent or close to the ampulla of the semicircular canal (cupulolithiasis). In cases of canalithiasis, the nystagmus beats toward the affected ear when the head is rolled to the affected side (geotropic nystagmus). When the head is rotated toward the unaffected side, the direction of the nystagmus changes to beat toward the unaffected side (geotropic). In cases of cupulolithiasis, the direction of nystagmus is away from the affected side (ageotropic) when the head is turned toward the affected side and again reverses direction when the head is rotated toward the unaffected side (ageotropic). The nystagmus and vertigo are typically less intense when the head is turned toward the unaffected side. Additional maneuvers may be used to determine the affected ear in horizontal canal BPPV [25].

The midline head-hang maneuver is used to diagnose BPPV of either superior semicircular canal. The patient is seated on an examination table with head upright and in the midline. The patient is then moved rapidly to the supine position with the head hanging approximately 90° below the horizontal plane. A positive test elicits downbeating nystagmus, often with a torsional component.

Treatment for BPPV involves canalith repositioning maneuvers specific to each canal. Posterior canal BPPV is typically treated with the Epley maneuver. Alternatively, the Semont or Brandt-Daroff maneuvers may be used. Horizontal canal BPPV is treated with the Barbecue Roll or Gufoni maneuvers. Superior canal BPPV can be treated with a variety of maneuvers, including the modified deep Brandt-Daroff maneuver, Yacavino maneuver, and standing inversion maneuver. Videos demonstrating exam and repositioning maneuvers are available online accompanying prior publications [19, 24].

Most patients experience symptom relief from one or two treatment maneuvers. However, canalith repositioning maneuvers may result in conversion of BPPV to another canal. BPPV can also reoccur in the same or other canals. Thus, some patients require repeated treatments which can be performed by a clinician, in vestibular physical therapy or at home. BPPV may also resolve without treatment. For rare cases of multiply recurrent BPPV, more definitive treatment may be considered including posterior semicircular canal occlusion, singular neurectomy, or vestibular neurectomy, though such interventions are very rarely indicated in the pediatric population.

There is an increased risk of BPPV among patients with migraine that has been reported among both pediatric and adult patients [1, 23, 26–28]. These disorders may also occur in a triad along with persistent postural-perceptual dizziness (PPPD) [1]. Head trauma can result in the development of both migraine and BPPV. Pathophysiologic mechanisms for the co-occurrence of BPPV and migraine in patients without head trauma are otherwise not well established. Patients with concurrent vestibular migraine and BPPV may respond well to repositioning maneuvers initially, but may experience frequent recurrences until their migraines are effectively managed [23, 29].

Vestibular migraine can also frequently cause positional nystagmus that can mimic BPPV, which is referred to as central positional nystagmus [29–31]. Characteristics that may help to differentiate central positional nystagmus from BPPV are summarized in Fig. 7.6. It should also be noted that patients with vestibular migraine are more prone to experiencing dizziness in gravity dependent head positions than non-migraineurs. Central positional nystagmus can also occur in the setting of posterior fossa masses or congenital anomalies, such as a Chiari malformation, so brain imaging should be considered when the clinical history is atypical for vestibular migraine.

7.2.2 Persistent Postural-Perceptual Dizziness

Persistent postural-perceptual dizziness (PPPD) is a functional neurological disorder (FND) that was established as a diagnosis in 2017, replacing past functional dizziness diagnoses including phobic postural vertigo, space-motion discomfort, visual vertigo, and chronic subjective dizziness [32]. PPPD is a chronic disorder characterized by dizziness, unsteadiness or non-spinning vertigo, on most days for at least 3 months. Symptoms are exacerbated by upright posture, active or passive movement, and exposure to moving or complex visual stimuli. It develops following an initial insult or disorder that causes dizziness or imbalance, such as peripheral and central vestibular disorders, psychological distress or other medical illness.

1. Clinical history is atypical for BPPV
2. Dizziness occurs in multiple/all diagnostic maneuver positions, despite nystagmus only occurring in selected positions
3. Nystagmus occurs in multiple/all positions (often with a similar pattern), despite vertigo only occurring in selected positions
4. Dizziness with diagnostic maneuvers is non-vertiginous and vague in character
5. Dizziness symptoms may occur in different positions than those that trigger nystagmus
6. Nystagmus patterns are inconsistent with what would be expected from the semicircular canal associated with that specific diagnostic maneuver
7. Nystagmus has a predominantly vertical component without torsion
8. Symptoms persist for several minutes after returning to neutral head/body position
9. Positional nystagmus and/or positional dizziness does not resolve after multiple treatment maneuvers
10. Nystagmus pattern suggests multiple canal and/or bilateral involvement

Fig. 7.6 Features distinguishing central positional nystagmus from BPPV

Patients with PPPD experience significant distress and/or functional impairment with days out of school or work. In one large series, 43% of children were out of school or in school part time at the time of diagnosis [33]. Diagnostic criteria, defined by the Bárány Society in the International Classification of Vestibular Disorders are included in Fig. 7.7 [34].

Of pediatric patients with dizziness and/or imbalance seen at a large tertiary care center, 7.3% were diagnosed with PPPD [33]. Among pediatric patients, it occurs most commonly in teenagers with a female predominance. PPPD frequently co-occurs with diagnoses like vestibular migraine and BPPV (Fig. 7.8). Overlapping symptoms of chronic migraine and PPPD sometimes obscures diagnosis. It is important for clinicians to remain vigilant in looking for overlapping and concurrent diagnoses in this population.

The pathophysiology of PPPD is not definitively established, however, it is understood as an FND which develops due to a central process involving maladaptive compensatory strategies that are maintained following an initial vestibular insult. Compensatory strategies including stiffened posture and a shift toward reliance on visual input over vestibular input may be helpful in the immediate aftermath of a vestibular insult but become maladaptive when maintained longer term. In PPPD, chronic dizziness is maintained by unhelpful appraisals, activity and stimulus avoidance, safety behaviors, abnormal (stiffened) postural control, over-attention to body sensations, and over-reliance on visual stimuli [32]. Neurotic personality traits and anxiety are highly prevalent and may predispose patients to developing PPPD. A chronic physiological anxiety (sympathetic nervous system) response is

A. One or more symptoms of dizziness, unsteadiness, or non-spinning vertigo are present on most days for 3 months or more.
    1. Symptoms last for prolonged (hours-long) periods of time, but may wax and wane in severity.
    2. Symptoms need not be present continuously throughout the entire day.
B. Persistent symptoms occur without specific provocation, but are exacerbated by three factors:
    1. Upright posture
    2. Active or passive motion without regard to direction or position, and
    3. Exposure to moving visual stimuli or complex visual patterns.
C. The disorder is precipitated by conditions that cause vertigo, unsteadiness, dizziness, or problems with balance including acute, episodic, or chronic vestibular syndromes, other neurologic or medical illnesses, or psychological distress.
    1. When the precipitant is an acute or episodic condition, symptoms settle into the pattern of criterion A as the precipitant resolves, but they may occur intermittently at first, and then consolidate into a persistent course.
    2. When the precipitant is a chronic syndrome, symptoms may develop slowly at first and worsen gradually.
D. Symptoms cause significant distress or functional impairment.
E. Symptoms are not better accounted for by another disease or disorder.

Fig. 7.7 Persistent postural-perceptual dizziness diagnostic criteria

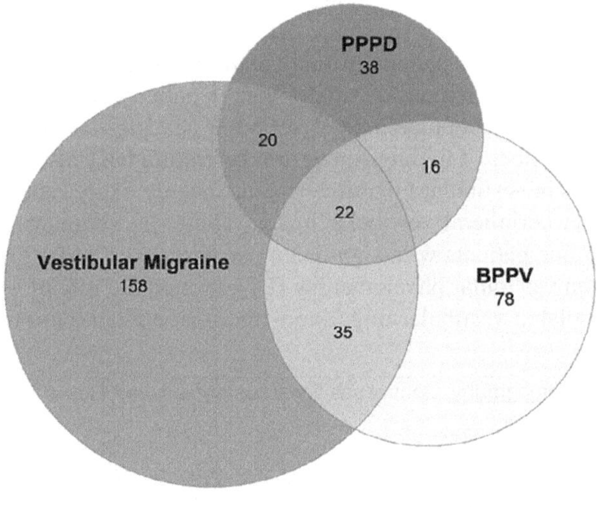

Fig. 7.8 Concurrent vestibular migraine, persistent postural-perceptual dizziness (PPPD), and benign paroxysmal positional vertigo (BPPV) among non-post concussion patients (n = 757). Reprinted with permission from Wang et al. 2021 [1]

ubiquitous in patients with chronic dizziness, and addressing this component plays an essential role in PPPD management.

Treatment of PPPD begins with deliberate counseling regarding the diagnosis and treatment plan, which involves vestibular physical therapy, cognitive behavioral therapy (CBT), and/or selective serotonin reuptake inhibitor (SSRI) or serotonin and norepinephrine reuptake inhibitor (SNRI) medication. Management of concurrent diagnoses, including vestibular migraine, is critical as well. Recovery takes months to years, but 85% of patients in one series reported resolution of constant dizziness at most recent follow-up [33].

Similar to the issues described above with BPPV, it should be noted that vestibular migraine symptoms can also be chronic, with interictal features between symptom flares such as head motion sensitivity, postural dizziness, disequilibrium, and/or visual flow intolerance, all of which can mimic concurrent PPPD [35]. Thus, it is paramount that any suspected migrainous component be adequately addressed in treating patients with suspected PPPD before pursuing more PPPD-specific interventions, such as vestibular physiotherapy with systematic desensitization (habituation) therapy and SSRI/SNRI medications. SNRI medications and CBT may be effective in treating vestibular migraine, in addition to treating PPPD, so these treatments can be considered right away for patients with suspected concurrent VM + PPPD [36, 37].

7.2.3 Vestibular Loss

Peripheral vestibular loss has been shown to occur relatively frequently in vestibular migraine patients, particularly in adults, though the rates and degree of vestibular loss in vestibular migraine patients varies greatly between studies. In general, the degree of vestibular loss is typically milder than in patients with primary peripheral vestibulopathies (e.g., vestibulotoxicity, vestibular neuritis, labyrinthitis, Ménière's disease, etc.). A number of findings on vestibular testing have also been reported to be more common in vestibular migraine patients that are likely central in origin and not due to direct peripheral vestibular losses. These are summarized in Fig. 7.9. Vestibular migraine patients with significant peripheral vestibular losses on testing may benefit from vestibular physiotherapy (PT), though the role of vestibular PT in the setting of isolated vestibular migraine without significant peripheral vestibular

1. Videonystagmography: Central positional nystagmus (see Figure 6 above) and/or spontaneous nystagmus
2. Caloric testing: Abnormal unilateral weakness score and/or directional preponderance score
3. Rotary chair: Reduced gain, phase lag, and/or increased time constant
4. Subjective visual vertical: Abnormal deviation of perceived vertical
5. Vestibular evoked myogenic potential testing: Reduced or absent responses
6. Video head impulse testing: Reduced gain

Fig. 7.9 Vestibular test findings reported to occur with increased frequency in Vestibular Migraine Patients [29, 39–42]

impairment is likely low [38]. The mechanism of peripheral vestibular loss in vestibular migraine has not been definitively established, but likely shares overlap with the pathophysiologic mechanisms of recurrent BPPV and of sensorineural hearing loss in vestibular migraine patients.

7.3 Non-Vestibular Conditions Associated with Migraine

The following non-vestibular conditions frequently occur concurrently in children and adolescents with vestibular migraine and may cause symptoms that overlap with or mimic vestibular migraine symptoms, such as dizziness, vision changes, and/or headache. Addressing these conditions is often an important component of effective vestibular migraine management.

7.3.1 Dysautonomia

Dysautonomia results from dysregulation of the autonomic nervous system. Various types of dysautonomia, including hemodynamic intolerance, vasovagal syncope and postural orthostatic tachycardia syndrome (POTS), are common in pediatric patients. Patients with hemodynamic intolerance most often describe lightheadedness during upright positioning, though dizziness or vertigo may be described [43]. Associated symptoms can include tachycardia, palpitations, tinnitus, visual disturbance (e.g., tunnel vision or graying of vision), paresthesias, nausea, fatigue, cognitive deficits, abdominal discomfort, headache, and photophobia. Diagnostic testing is typically performed with tilt table and/or orthostatic blood pressure and heart rate testing. Diagnosis of POTS is made in patients with 3 months or more of symptoms and excessive upright tachycardia in the absence of orthostatic hypotension during standing testing. Diagnostic criteria include an increase in heart rate of at least 30 beats per min in adults, and 40 beats per min for adolescents aged 12–19 years, or an increase in heart rate to >120 beats per min, in the first ten minutes of upright position without a decrease in systolic blood pressure > 20 mm Hg [44]. Treatment of POTS includes non-pharmacologic interventions including optimizing hydration and salt intake, physical therapy, and use of compression stockings and a variety of pharmacologic treatments (e.g., midodrine, fludrocortisone, propranolol, etc.) aimed at supporting blood pressure and/or heart rate elevation. Pharmacologic management is discussed in detail elsewhere [45].

Migraine often co-occurs with dysautonomia, and in particular, with POTS. As noted above, this is likely due, at least in part, to the ubiquitous sympathetic nervous system upregulation in patients with chronic dizziness and/or pain. Demographic features are similar among both conditions. Like migraine, onset of POTS in pediatric patients typically occurs in adolescence. There is a strong female predominance in both conditions, and both are more common in Caucasian individuals [46, 47]. Migraine and POTS share common triggers for disease onset including infection and concussion [48]. Symptoms of both disorders may be triggered or exacerbated by dehydration, illness, and exertion. Both conditions are also associated with anxiety and depression [49, 50]. Ideally, the term POTS should be reserved for patients who present with the condition as an isolated primary phenomenon, while a POTS presentation from autonomic dysfunction that is secondary to another condition, such as (e.g. anxiety, migraine, PPPD, concussion, etc.) should be labeled under the umbrella of dysautonomia.

There are overlapping symptoms that make dysautonomia difficult to diagnose among patients with migraine. Symptoms of headache, nausea, lightheadedness or dizziness and fatigue are common symptoms in both conditions. Diagnosis requires a thorough history, exam, and attention to the possibility of multiple coexisting pathologies. Some treatments for dysautonomia overlap with treatments for vestibular migraine, including hydration, increased physical activity, beta-blockers and CBT. In patients with concurrent dysautonomia and vestibular migraine, it is likely that their autonomic dysfunction will improve once dizziness and headache symptoms are better controlled with migraine therapies.

7.3.2 Concussion

An association between concussion and migraine has been established among athletes [51]. Migraine often develops following concussion, with 15–33% of patients with sports-related concussion reported to develop post-traumatic migraine. Development of post-traumatic migraine is associated with worse impairment and prolonged recovery from concussion [52, 53]. Additionally, migraine may predispose to concussion. Concussion and migraine have shared pathophysiologic mechanisms, including trigeminal system activation, cortical spreading depression, and failure in brain ion homeostasis [54]. Overlapping symptoms make accurate diagnosis challenging and can lead to inappropriate or inadequate treatment. Most of the other conditions outlined in this section that often co-occur with vestibular migraine are also relatively common following concussion, including BPPV, autonomic dysfunction, anxiety, peripheral vestibular loss, PPPD/FND, and temporomandibular dysfunction (TMD).

7.3.3 Anxiety and Depression

Anxiety and depressive disorders are more common among children and adolescents with migraine compared to healthy peers. Often, anxiety and depression are secondary, arising in the setting of distressing physical symptoms. In a large meta-analysis, the odds of anxiety and depressive disorders was about two times higher among pediatric patients with migraine compared to controls [50]. Pediatric patients with migraine have a higher tendency toward internalizing symptoms, which is the tendency to react to stress with internal processes such as anxiety, somatization and depression [55, 56]. The tendency toward internalizing symptoms in response to pain may lead to cognitive, affective, and behavioral factors such as poor sleep, withdrawal from activities, negativity bias and attention bias, that in turn contribute to the development or maintenance of both psychiatric and migraine disorders [50, 57]. Additional theories have been proposed regarding the link between psychiatric comorbidities and migraine including exposure to environmental adversity and shared hormonal, biochemical, and genetic factors.

Importantly, the presence of internalizing disorders (depression and anxiety) is associated with poorer migraine outcomes including higher headache frequency and lower quality of life [58–61].

It is important for pediatric migraine providers to screen for anxiety and depression. Validated questionnaires may be used.

Treatment for pediatric patients with anxiety in the setting of vestibular migraine may include conventional talk therapy, CBT, biofeedback, dialectical behavioral therapy (DBT), and/or medication (SSRIs, SNRIs, beta-blockers, and less commonly, tricyclic antidepressants). Benzodiazepines may be used short term for severe symptoms but should be avoided in the long term, particularly in pediatric patients.

7.3.4 Temporomandibular Dysfunction

TMD refers to myofascial pain and tension within the masticatory muscles (e.g., temporalis, masseter, pterygoids, etc.) often concurrently with inflammation of the temporomandibular joint (TMJ). TMD symptoms are associated with migraine, as well as increased migraine frequency and medication use [62, 63]. The exact mechanism of this relationship is unknown, but most likely results from chronically increased sympathetic nervous system activation in patients with chronic dizziness and/or chronic pain, as described in the above sections. Patients with TMD will often experience headaches in a temporal distribution, which may be misdiagnosed as migraine flares. Jaw-specific symptoms may be present, including pain with chewing and audible/palpable TMJ clicking or popping. Otologic symptoms are also often present, including tinnitus, aural fullness, and otalgia, which may result in concurrent TMD and vestibular migraine being misdiagnosed as Ménière's disease. Examination for TMD can be performed at the bedside by checking for tenderness to palpation of the TMJ joints with jaw opening/closing (both intra-aurally with the examiner's finger pushing gently against the anterior surface of the lateral ear canal and extra-aurally with the examiner's finger placed just anterior to the tragus), as well as by checking for tenderness of the masseter muscle by palpating behind the mandibular ramus bilaterally and on the anterior surface of the ramus intra-orally with a gloved hand. Treatments for TMD can include a sustained course of standing non-steroidal anti-inflammatory drug therapy (e.g., naproxen or ibuprofen) for 1–2 weeks, a course of a soft, non-chewing diet (usually also for 1–2 weeks), a nightguard, physiotherapy, Botox injections, and rarely surgery. Treating TMD in migraineurs may help to reduce baseline pain symptoms and triggering of migraine flares, but this has yet to be demonstrated in quality, peer-reviewed studies.

7.3.5 Motion Sickness

Motion sickness occurs during and/or after exposure to real or perceived motion, such as in a car, boat, amusement park rides, or virtual reality games. Though occasional motion sickness is common among the general population, a subset of patients experiences severe motion sickness, which has a significant impact on quality of life [64, 65]. Motion sickness is prevalent and can affect children of all ages, including infants [66]. Similar to migraine, motion sickness is more common in females than in males [67]. Motion sickness is extremely common in patients with migraine, occurring in at least half of migraine sufferers [68, 69].

In addition to shared demographic features, migraine and motion sickness share overlapping symptoms including nausea, fatigue, and headache. Motion sensitivity is also associated with upper abdominal symptoms, cold sweat, increased salivation, and pallor [70]. Pathophysiologic links have been proposed including shared neural circuitry and neurotransmitters [71].

Genetic predisposition has been established for both migraine and motion sensitivity, though it is uncertain if these are shared. Both conditions are influenced by hormones, with increased susceptibility to both migraine and motion sickness occurring during females' menstrual cycles [72].

The senior author has anecdotally observed a significant number of very young children with an early onset severe predilection to motion sickness in the absence of other migraine symptoms that have gone on to develop vestibular migraine later in childhood, often accompanied by a reduction in motion sickness symptoms. This could suggest that early onset severe motion sickness in very young children could represent a migraine variant, in and of itself, though this possibility requires further investigation.

Treatment for motion sickness includes behavioral interventions, vestibular physical therapy, and/or medication. Dramamine (dimenhydrinate), Benadryl (diphenhydramine), ondansetron, and meclizine may be used as needed prior to exposure. Patients with severe and/or frequent symptoms typically benefit greatly from treatment with daily cyproheptadine, which is a medication that is often used for migraine prevention in young children [66]. Although cyproheptadine is an antihistamine, its efficacy for migraine disorders and for motion sickness likely occur by its additional pharmacological antagonism of 5-HT_2 receptors.

7.3.6 Hearing Loss

A link between sensorineural hearing loss (SNHL) and migraine has been reported among adult patients. There is an increased risk of SNHL and sudden SNHL among adult patients with migraine [73–75]. Additionally, a subset of migraine patients experience fluctuating hearing loss and aural fullness in association with migraine, which has been labeled cochlear migraine [76]. Hearing loss can affect quality of life in patients who are already suffering from migraine and should be identified and addressed when present. While this association has not been established in pediatric patients with migraine, this emerging data warrants future study in the pediatric population.

Take-Home Points

- Pediatric migraine variants with vestibular symptoms can include BPTI, RVC/BPVC, vestibular migraine of childhood, and cyclical vomiting.
- Conditions that can frequently co-occur with or mimic vestibular migraine include BPPV, PPPD, peripheral vestibulopathy, autonomic dysfunction, anxiety, depression, concussion, TMD, motion sickness, and hearing loss.
- Given that vestibular migraine and its variants are collectively the most common cause of vertigo in children, and that vestibular migraine can often mimic many of these conditions, it is important to strongly consider migraine as a major factor in any child or adolescent presenting with vertigo before considering other alternative causes.
- Treating concurrent conditions that can exacerbate vestibular migraine symptoms—such as anxiety, autonomic dysfunction, BPPV, and TMD—may help to reduce direct migraine symptomatology, as well.
- Cyproheptadine can often be an effective preventative therapy for many vestibular migraine variants in young children, including BPTI, RVC/BPVC, vestibular migraine, cyclical vomiting, and motion sickness.
- Management of anxiety and/or autonomic dysfunction with psychological therapies and/or medications may be helpful for vestibular migraine, both directly and indirectly.
- Although vestibular migraine is a clinical diagnosis, a number of abnormalities can often be seen on vestibular testing that can support a migraine diagnosis while also mimicking other vestibulopathies, such as BPPV and vestibular loss.

References

1. Wang A, Zhou G, Lipson S, Kawai K, Corcoran M, Brodsky JR. Multifactorial characteristics of pediatric dizziness and imbalance. Laryngoscope. 2021;131(4):E1308–14.
2. Rosman NP, Douglass LM, Sharif UM, Paolini J. The neurology of benign paroxysmal torticollis of infancy: report of 10 new cases and review of the literature. J Child Neurol. 2009;24(2):155–60.
3. Brodsky J, Kaur K, Shoshany T, Lipson S, Zhou G. Benign paroxysmal migraine variants of infancy and childhood: transitions and clinical features. Eur J Paediatr Neurol. 2018;22(4):667–73.
4. Headache classification committee of the international headache society (ihs) the international classification of headache disorders, 3rd . Cephalalgia. 2018;38(1):1-211.
5. Al-Twaijri WA, Shevell MI. Pediatric migraine equivalents: occurrence and clinical features in practice. Pediatr Neurol. 2002;26(5):365–8.
6. Giffin NJ, Benton S, Goadsby PJ. Benign paroxysmal torticollis of infancy: four new cases and linkage to cacna1a mutation. Dev Med Child Neurol. 2002;44(7):490–3.

7. Shin M, Douglass LM, Milunsky JM, Rosman NP. The genetics of benign paroxysmal torticollis of infancy: is there an association with mutations in the cacna1a gene? J Child Neurol. 2016;31(8):1057–61.
8. Brodsky JR, Kaur K, Shoshany T, et al. Torticollis in children with enlarged vestibular aqueducts. Int J Pediatr Otorhinolaryngol. 2020;131:109862.
9. van de Berg R, Widdershoven J, Bisdorff A, et al. Vestibular migraine of childhood and recurrent vertigo of childhood: diagnostic criteria consensus document of the committee for the classification of vestibular disorders of the barany society and the international headache society. J Vestib Res. 2021;31(1):1–9.
10. Batuecas-Caletrio A, Martin-Sanchez V, Cordero-Civantos C, et al. Is benign paroxysmal vertigo of childhood a migraine precursor? Eur J Paediatr Neurol. 2013;17(4):397–400.
11. Lanzi G, Balottin U, Fazzi E, Tagliasacchi M, Manfrin M, Mira E. Benign paroxysmal vertigo of childhood: a long-term follow-up. Cephalalgia. 1994;14(6):458–60.
12. Krams B, Echenne B, Leydet J, Rivier F, Roubertie A. Benign paroxysmal vertigo of childhood: long-term outcome. Cephalalgia. 2011;31(4):439–43.
13. Lindskog U, Odkvist L, Noaksson L, Wallquist J. Benign paroxysmal vertigo in childhood: a long-term follow-up. Headache. 1999;39(1):33–7.
14. Frazier R, Li BUK, Venkatesan T. Diagnosis and management of cyclic vomiting syndrome: a critical review. Am J Gastroenterol. 2023;118(7):1157–67.
15. Lagman-Bartolome AM, Lay C. Pediatric migraine variants: a review of epidemiology, diagnosis, treatment, and outcome. Curr Neurol Neurosci Rep. 2015;15(6):34.
16. Benninga MA, Faure C, Hyman PE, St James Roberts I, Schechter NL, Nurko S. Childhood functional gastrointestinal disorders: Neonate/toddler. Gastroenterology. 2016; 15:S0016-5085(16):00182–7.
17. Hyams JS, Di Lorenzo C, Saps M, Shulman RJ, Staiano A, van Tilburg M. Functional disorders: children and adolescents. Gastroenterology. 2016;15:S0016-5085(16):00181–5.
18. Stanghellini V, Chan FK, Hasler WL, et al. Gastroduodenal disorders. Gastroenterology. 2016;150(6):1380–92.
19. Wang A, Zhou G, Kawai K, O'Brien M, Shearer AE, Brodsky JR. Benign paroxysmal positional vertigo in children and adolescents with concussion. Sports Health. 2021;13(4):380–6.
20. O'Reilly RC, Morlet T, Nicholas BD, et al. Prevalence of vestibular and balance disorders in children. Otol Neurotol. 2010;31(9):1441–4.
21. Lee JD, Kim CH, Hong SM, et al. Prevalence of vestibular and balance disorders in children and adolescents according to age: a multi-center study. Int J Pediatr Otorhinolaryngol. 2017;94:36–9.
22. Wiener-Vacher SR, Quarez J, Priol AL. Epidemiology of vestibular impairments in a pediatric population. Semin Hear. 2018;39(3):229–42.
23. Brodsky JR, Lipson S, Wilber J, Zhou G. Benign paroxysmal positional vertigo (bppv) in children and adolescents: clinical features and response to therapy in 110 pediatric patients. Otol Neurotol. 2018;39(3):344–50.
24. Kim JS, Zee DS. Clinical practice. Benign paroxysmal positional vertigo. N Engl J Med. 2014;370(12):1138–47.
25. Bhattacharyya N, Gubbels SP, Schwartz SR, et al. Clinical practice guideline: Benign paroxysmal positional vertigo (update). Otolaryngol Head Neck Surg. 2017;156(3_suppl):S1–S47.
26. von Brevern M, Radtke A, Lezius F, et al. Epidemiology of benign paroxysmal positional vertigo: a population based study. J Neurol Neurosurg Psychiatry. 2007;78(7):710–5.
27. Teixido M, Baker A, Isildak H. Migraine and benign paroxysmal positional vertigo: a single-institution review. J Laryngol Otol. 2017;131(6):508–13.
28. Yetiser S, Gokmen MH. Clinical aspects of benign paroxysmal positional vertigo associated with migraine. Int Tinnitus J. 2015;19(2):64–8.
29. Tian E, Li F, Liu D, et al. Dispelling mist that obscures positional vertigo in vestibular migraine. Brain Sci. 2023;13:10.
30. Lemos J, Strupp M. Central positional nystagmus: an update. J Neurol. 2022;269(4):1851–60.
31. El-Badry MM, Samy H, Kabel AM, Rafat FM, Sanyelbhaa H. Clinical criteria of positional vertical nystagmus in vestibular migraine. Acta Otolaryngol. 2017;137(7):720–2.

32. Popkirov S, Staab JP, Stone J. Persistent postural-perceptual dizziness (pppd): a common, characteristic and treatable cause of chronic dizziness. Pract Neurol. 2018;18(1):5–13.
33. Wang A, Fleischman KM, Kawai K, Corcoran M, Brodsky JR. Persistent postural-perceptual dizziness in children and adolescents. Otol Neurotol. 2021;42(8):e1093–100.
34. Staab JP, Eckhardt-Henn A, Horii A, et al. Diagnostic criteria for persistent postural-perceptual dizziness (pppd): consensus document of the committee for the classification of vestibular disorders of the barany society. J Vestib Res. 2017;27(4):191–208.
35. Tarnutzer AA, Kaski D. What's in a name? Chronic vestibular migraine or persistent postural perceptual dizziness? Brain Sci. 2023;13:12.
36. Webster KE, Dor A, Galbraith K, et al. Non-pharmacological interventions for prophylaxis of vestibular migraine. Cochrane Database Syst Rev. 2023;4(4):CD015321.
37. Salviz M, Yuce T, Acar H, Karatas A, Acikalin RM. Propranolol and venlafaxine for vestibular migraine prophylaxis: a randomized controlled trial. Laryngoscope. 2016;126(1):169–74.
38. Alghadir AH, Anwer S. Effects of vestibular rehabilitation in the management of a vestibular migraine: a review. Front Neurol. 2018;9:440.
39. Young AS, Nham B, Bradshaw AP, et al. Clinical, oculographic, and vestibular test characteristics of vestibular migraine. Cephalalgia. 2021;41(10):1039–52.
40. Kang WS, Lee SH, Yang CJ, Ahn JH, Chung JW, Park HJ. Vestibular function tests for vestibular migraine: clinical implication of video head impulse and caloric tests. Front Neurol. 2016;7:166.
41. Li F, Xu J, Li GR, et al. The value of subjective visual vertical in diagnosis of vestibular migraine. Curr Med Sci. 2021;41(4):654–60.
42. Wu Y, Ling X, Song N, et al. Comparison of clinical characteristics and vestibular function test results in patients with vestibular migraine and meniere's disease. Braz J Otorhinolaryngol. 2023;89(4):101274.
43. Kim HA, Bisdorff A, Bronstein AM, et al. Hemodynamic orthostatic dizziness/vertigo: diagnostic criteria. J Vestib Res. 2019;29(2-3):45–56.
44. Stewart JM, Boris JR, Chelimsky G, et al. Pediatric disorders of orthostatic intolerance. Pediatrics. 2018;141:1.
45. Miller AJ, Raj SR. Pharmacotherapy for postural tachycardia syndrome. Auton Neurosci. 2018;215:28–36.
46. Boris JR, Bernadzikowski T. Demographics of a large paediatric postural orthostatic tachycardia syndrome program. Cardiol Young. 2018;28(5):668–74.
47. Stewart WF, Lipton RB, Liberman J. Variation in migraine prevalence by race. Neurology. 1996;47(1):52–9.
48. Boris JR. Postural orthostatic tachycardia syndrome in children and adolescents. Auton Neurosci. 2018;215:97–101.
49. Moon J, Kim DY, Byun JI, et al. Orthostatic intolerance symptoms are associated with depression and diminished quality of life in patients with postural tachycardia syndrome. Health Qual Life Outcomes. 2016;14(1):144.
50. Falla K, Kuziek J, Mahnaz SR, Noel M, Ronksley PE, Orr SL. Anxiety and depressive symptoms and disorders in children and adolescents with migraine: a systematic review and meta-analysis. JAMA Pediatr. 2022;176(12):1176–87.
51. Eckner JT, Seifert T, Pescovitz A, Zeiger M, Kutcher JS. Is migraine headache associated with concussion in athletes? A case-control study. Clin J Sport Med. 2017;27(3):266–70.
52. Kontos AP, Elbin RJ, Lau B, et al. Posttraumatic migraine as a predictor of recovery and cognitive impairment after sport-related concussion. Am J Sports Med. 2013;41(7):1497–504.
53. Mihalik JP, Register-Mihalik J, Kerr ZY, Marshall SW, McCrea MC, Guskiewicz KM. Recovery of posttraumatic migraine characteristics in patients after mild traumatic brain injury. Am J Sports Med. 2013;41(7):1490–6.
54. Seifert T. The relationship of migraine and other headache disorders to concussion. Handb Clin Neurol. 2018;158:119–26.

55. Dresler T, Caratozzolo S, Guldolf K, et al. Understanding the nature of psychiatric comorbidity in migraine: a systematic review focused on interactions and treatment implications. J Headache Pain. 2019;20(1):51.
56. Balottin U, Fusar Poli P, Termine C, Molteni S, Galli F. Psychopathological symptoms in child and adolescent migraine and tension-type headache: a meta-analysis. Cephalalgia. 2013;33(2):112–22.
57. Vinall J, Pavlova M, Asmundson GJ, Rasic N, Noel M. Mental health comorbidities in pediatric chronic pain: a narrative review of epidemiology, models, neurobiological mechanisms and treatment. Children (Basel). 2016;3:4.
58. Vannatta K, Getzoff EA, Powers SW, Noll RB, Gerhardt CA, Hershey AD. Multiple perspectives on the psychological functioning of children with and without migraine. Headache. 2008;48(7):994–1004.
59. Cooper PJ, Bawden HN, Camfield PR, Camfield CS. Anxiety and life events in childhood migraine. Pediatrics. 1987;79(6):999–1004.
60. Orr SL, Turner A, Kabbouche MA, et al. Predictors of short-term prognosis while in pediatric headache care: an observational study. Headache. 2019;59(4):543–55.
61. Heckman BD, Holroyd KA, Himawan L, et al. Do psychiatric comorbidities influence headache treatment outcomes? Results of a naturalistic longitudinal treatment study. Pain. 2009;146(1-2):56–64.
62. Fernandes G, Arruda MA, Bigal ME, Camparis CM, Goncalves DAG. Painful temporomandibular disorder is associated with migraine in adolescents: a case-control study. J Pain. 2019;20(10):1155–63.
63. Ashraf J, Zaproudina N, Suominen AL, Sipila K, Narhi M, Saxlin T. Association between temporomandibular disorders pain and migraine: results of the health 2000 survey. J Oral Facial Pain Headache. 2019;33(4):399–407.
64. Lee SH, Jeong SH, Kim JS, et al. Effect of prophylactic medication on associated dizziness and motion sickness in migraine. Otol Neurotol. 2018;39(1):e45–51.
65. Henriques IF, Douglas de Oliveira DW, Oliveira-Ferreira F, Andrade PM. Motion sickness prevalence in school children. Eur J Pediatr. 2014;173(11):1473–82.
66. Lipson S, Wang A, Corcoran M, Zhou G, Brodsky JR. Severe motion sickness in infants and children. Eur J Paediatr Neurol. 2020;28:176–9.
67. Turner M, Griffin MJ, Holland I. Airsickness and aircraft motion during short-haul flights. Aviat Space Environ Med. 2000;71(12):1181–9.
68. Kayan A, Hood JD. Neuro-otological manifestations of migraine. Brain. 1984;107(Pt 4):1123–42.
69. Baloh RW. Neurotology of migraine. Headache. 1997;37(10):615–21.
70. Graybiel A, Wood CD, Miller EF, Cramer DB. Diagnostic criteria for grading the severity of acute motion sickness. Aerosp Med. 1968;39(5):453–5.
71. Cuomo-Granston A, Drummond PD. Migraine and motion sickness: what is the link? Prog Neurobiol. 2010;91(4):300–12.
72. Grunfeld E, Gresty MA. Relationship between motion sickness, migraine and menstruation in crew members of a "round the world" yacht race. Brain Res Bull. 1998;47(5):433–6.
73. Guo Z, Wang J, Liu D, et al. Early detection and monitoring of hearing loss in vestibular migraine: extended high-frequency hearing. Front Aging Neurosci. 2022;14:1090322.
74. Mohammadi M, Taziki Balajelini MH, Rajabi A. Migraine and risk of sudden sensorineural hearing loss: a systematic review and meta-analysis. Laryngoscope Investig Otolaryngol. 2020;5(6):1089–95.
75. Campello CP, Lemos CAA, Andrade WTL, Melo LPF, Nunes GRS, Cavalcanti HG. Migraine associated with tinnitus and hearing loss in adults: a systematic review. Int J Audiol. 2024;63(1):1–7.
76. Benjamin T, Gillard D, Abouzari M, Djalilian HR, Sharon JD. Vestibular and auditory manifestations of migraine. Curr Opin Neurol. 2022;35(1):84–9.

GPSR Compliance

The European Union's (EU) General Product Safety Regulation (GPSR) is a set of rules that requires consumer products to be safe and our obligations to ensure this.

If you have any concerns about our products, you can contact us on ProductSafety@springernature.com

In case Publisher is established outside the EU, the EU authorized representative is:

Springer Nature Customer Service Center GmbH
Europaplatz 3
69115 Heidelberg, Germany

Batch number: 10738117

Printed by Printforce, the Netherlands